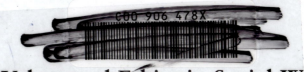

Culture, Values and Ethics in Social Work

This groundbreaking book examines the ways in which questions of culture and diversity impact on the values and ethics of social work. Using detailed case studies to illustrate key points for practice, Richard Hugman discusses how social workers can develop cross-cultural engagement in practice and work creatively with the tensions it sometimes involves.

Debates rage over whether there is a core set of unchangeable social work values or whether they might be different at different times and for different people. This textbook proposes a new approach of 'ethical pluralism' for social work practice, in which both shared humanity and the rich variety of cultures contribute to a more dynamic way of understanding social work's underpinning values and ethics. In particular, this book explores the implications of a pluralist approach to ethics for the central questions of:

- Human rights and social justice.
- Caring relationships.
- Social and personal responsibilities.
- Agency and autonomy.
- Values such as truth, honesty, openness, service and competence.

It is vital that social workers understand the values and ethics of their profession as a crucial part of the foundations on which practice is built and this is the only text to explore the connections between culture, values and ethics and fully develop the pluralist approach in social work. *Culture, Values and Ethics in Social Work* is essential reading for all social work students and academics.

Richard Hugman is Professor of Social Work at the University of New South Wales, Australia. He is also the Chair of the Permanent Committee on Ethics of the International Federation of Social Workers.

Culture, Values and Ethics in Social Work

Embracing diversity

Richard Hugman

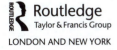
Routledge
Taylor & Francis Group

LONDON AND NEW YORK

First published 2013
by Routledge
2 Park Square, Milton Park, Abingdon, Oxon OX14 4RN

Simultaneously published in the USA and Canada
by Routledge
711 Third Avenue, New York, NY 10017

*Routledge is an imprint of the Taylor & Francis Group, an
informa business*

British Library Cataloguing in Publication Data
A catalogue record for this book is available from the British
Library

Library of Congress Cataloging-in-Publication Data
Hugman, Richard. 1954–
Culture, values and ethics in social work: embracing diversity /
Richard Hugman.
1. Social service—Moral and ethical aspects. 2. Social workers—
Professional ethics. 3. Cultural pluralism. I. Title.
HV10.5.H8382012   2012012051
174'.9361—dc23

ISBN13: 978-0-415-67348-8 (hbk)
ISBN13: 978-0-415-67349-5 (pbk)
ISBN13: 978-0-203-09490-7 (ebk)

Typeset in Sabon by
Book Now Ltd, London

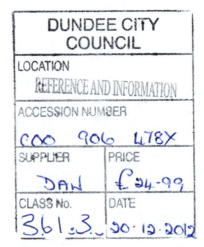

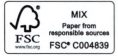

MIX
Paper from
responsible sources
FSC
www.fsc.org   FSC® C004839

Printed and bound in Great Britain by
TJ International Ltd, Padstow, Cornwall

Contents

Acknowledgements

The ideas and arguments presented in this book have developed over many years of practice, teaching and research in social work. In one sense to identify particular influences or assistance seems very difficult. However, there are a number of people to whom I owe thanks for challenges, encouragement, advice and help in avoiding some pitfalls. Conversations with colleagues in the International Federation of Social Workers have particularly stimulated my thinking (especially the members of the Permanent Committee on Ethics) – Laura Acotto, John Ang, Gary Bailey, Sarah Banks, Elaine Congress, Arne Groenningsaeter, David N. Jones, Charles Mbugua, Maria Moritz, Fiona Robertson and Ruth Stark. In another context I have been inspired by all of the many people with whom I have worked in Vietnam on the development of professional social work, most of all at UNICEF Vietnam – Le Hong Loan, Nguyen Thuy Hong, Vu Thi Le Thanh and the whole Child Protection Section – and at the University of Labour and Social Affairs – Bui Xuan Mai, Nguyen Thi Thai Lan and their colleagues. More broadly the development of this study has benefitted from many conversations with colleagues from many parts of the world, including Wendy Bowles, Vivienne Bozalek, Lesley Chenoweth, Lena Dominelli, Doug Durst, Mel Gray, Maria Harries, Tracie Mafile'o, Donna McAuliffe, Robyn Munford, Michael Reisch and Angie Yuen-Tsang. Closer to home, my colleagues in the Social Work group and the wider School of Social Sciences at the University of New South Wales provide the stimulating and supportive environment in which these ideas have grown. With regard to this study I would like to acknowledge the particular help and advice of Eileen Baldry, Linda Bartolomei, Jan Breckenridge, Mim Fox and Susan Green – and Sacha Kendall must be thanked for research assistance as well as for wide ranging debates about critical approaches to ethics. Although most may not even be aware of it, the continuing interaction with students over professional ethics and many other aspects of learning for professional practice constantly challenges my own thinking.

At Routledge Grace McInnes encouraged me to get started in the first place and both she and James Watson have provided editorial support and guidance throughout.

Finally, my greatest thanks are to Alex, whose constant love and care kept me going.

Richard Hugman
Sydney, May 2012

1 Introduction

Culture, values and ethics in social work and human services

Social welfare, social values and diversity

Practice in social work and the human services involves assisting a wide variety of people who require help in dealing with problems in their lives or otherwise providing social services to people so that they can live their lives more effectively. Children and their families, young people, people with physical or intellectual disabilities, with mental health needs, problems associated with old age, and issues faced by communities are all part of the broad focus of these services. Those who work in these services face complex and challenging issues that require careful thought and considerable skill in order to provide assistance appropriately. But in societies where people often have different ideas about what is good and what is right how should services be run and in what ways should people be assisted? These crucial questions are illustrated by the following hypothetical examples of practice. (All such examples in this book are hypothetical in that they do not describe any single actual situation – however, they are all drawn from the experience of the author or of practitioners from different parts of the world.)

> Julie is qualified as a teacher, Farouk in social work and Alan in youth and community work. They are the core staff of a youth service in a large city, providing a social centre and various forms of help to young people aged between 12 and 25. The neighbourhood where their youth centre is located is relatively poor and includes people whose family backgrounds are from Europe, Africa, the Caribbean, the Middle East, India, Pakistan and Hong Kong. Recently some of the young people have begun to ask for separate sessions for different ethnic groups because they are feeling that their cultural identities are being confronted by the attitudes and actions of other young people. This has now led to a particular situation where a young woman who wears *hijab* (a head scarf) is being taunted by those from other backgrounds, including some of the other young women. Julie, Farouk and Alan agree that the ethics of their different professions all support the right of this young woman to wear what is culturally appropriate for her, but they find that they are not agreed on whether there should be ethnic-specific sessions – Julie raises the point that if they create such a structure why should there not also be sessions specifically for young women. So although their

professions' ethics provide them with the ideas to think about this issue, it forces Julie, Farouk and Alan to recognize that these are not simply rules or instructions that can be applied as a technical solution. In the end they will have to make some difficult choices that relate ethics to questions of culture and difference.

In another part of the city the following situation is occurring.

> Imelda is employed by a small independent organization that provides social sup-port services to people with long-term ill-health and disabilities. Her role is to review direct everyday care services and to make changes to plans with service users when necessary. One of the families that Imelda is reviewing arrived in the country from South Asia about 22 years ago. The primary service user is a young woman, Gunawathie, aged 20, who has a degenerative disability and now requires constant care. In conversation with the family it becomes apparent to Imelda that neither Gunawathie nor her family are aware of how quickly she is likely to become more disabled or the likely length of her life. When Imelda checks with the family's doctor she is told that as the parents 'clearly' wanted to have hope for their daughter it was previously decided not to force the disclosure of this informa-tion. It is stated that the treating team considered this decision to be supported by the cultural expectations of the family. Imelda is aware that giving this informa-tion is widely accepted as the prerogative of the medical profession (and she does not have medical training) so she cannot make such a disclosure, but she feels uneasy that she is being asked to collude with the family and other professionals in withholding the truth of the situation from someone who is now an adult and who she regards as having a right to know the facts about her health.

In both these situations the values and ethics of those who are providing human ser-vices are central to the way in which they understand their role, the organizations that they work in and the choices that they face in their practice. But they are also faced with the challenge that not everyone agrees on what is the right thing to do. They have come up against the central question of a plural society: 'when is different sim-ply different and when is it wrong?' (Healy, 2007, p. 13). Julie, Farouk, Alan and Imelda all have to resolve this so that they can act and they have to do so as members of professional or occupational groups as well as employees of human service agen-cies. (This point is discussed further in Chapter 8.)

In all societies, throughout recorded human history, there have been recognized ways of providing assistance to individuals, families, groups and communities who have required help in dealing with problems and difficulties. Such arrangements can be understood as 'social welfare', in that they concern the social well-being of peo-ple as this is shaped by any given society. As societies have changed and developed, the form of such assistance has also changed, reflecting the institutions and values that predominate in any particular time and place. What is considered as 'well-being', or 'living well', differs between historical and cultural contexts. The 'right' way to assist those who face problems and difficulties in daily life is closely interwoven with politics, religion and other aspects of social structures in any given situation (Day, 2000). So in order to understand the field of social welfare it is necessary to consider institutions and practices in the context of the values held by members of a society.

Identifying values as a central feature of an analysis of social welfare immediately raises a number of other questions. Which values are central to social welfare? Are the values underpinning a concern with well-being shared throughout a society and, if not, whose values prevail? Moreover, when an international and historical perspective is taken, (how) can the differences between the values that can be observed at various times and in various places be understood as part of the same overall human concern with social well-being? Are they simply different ways of expressing the same human objective or should they be seen as separate activities that have only a superficial resemblance with each other? Such questions point to the necessity of examining variations between perspectives on social welfare that reflect a corresponding diversity of values concerning what should be done to promote social well-being and how this should be accomplished.

These are the underlying questions to which this book is addressed. It explores the significance of values as the basis of thinking about social work and human services, as the modern institutional response to social welfare issues, and connects this with the challenge that arises from the differences between cultures in considering what should be done to promote and assist the achievement of social well-being. Thus, social welfare is considered here as a matter of values before it is a question of institutional arrangements or practice techniques. In other words, *how* people seek to provide for social welfare comes from the ways in which well-being is seen. So ideas about the right ways to address social welfare have their foundation in beliefs and values about what is good.

The implication of this understanding for the practices and institutions of social welfare is that they are judged in terms of the goals that are set by values. Such a way of looking at this question reflects the old saying that '*form* follows *function*'. Yet function here is not simply a matter of technique, it concerns the goals of social welfare which, as already stated, embody those things that people regard as most important – in other words, they are based on values.

In the language of ethics, what is good or right about practices and institutions can only be judged in terms of their goals and not the other way around. However, this is not to suggest that ends justify all possible means. As discussed later in this book, means must be congruent with goals, otherwise they become contradictory. Practices and institutions also have to be understood in terms of values. Then, because values cannot be separated from questions of culture, the goals and practices of social welfare must be understood as embedded in culture.

So, in summary, the analysis presented in this book examines the dynamic connections between four main elements, namely culture, values, ethics, and social work and human services. Each of these elements is outlined in this chapter in order to provide the basis for the following discussion. In the following chapters more detailed questions are added to those already identified above. In what ways do the concerns of social work and human services relate to people's views of living well and of the good society? Where people disagree in their views about values are differences between such visions of human well-being reasonable? What are the implications of differences in values (goals) for thinking about social welfare institutions and practices (means)? How will answering these questions assist in the development of 'better' institutions and practices in social welfare?

Culture

The first of the four elements to this analysis is that of culture. This concept refers to the set of ideas and practices that are understood to constitute a society as a whole (Kuper, 1999; Eriksen, 2006). In this sense, culture is the shared values, attitudes and expectations that people who regard themselves as being of the same broad social grouping would see as characterizing what it is to be a member of that group. Culture is a combination of a 'world-view' and of social practices that express and sustain that view. So culture includes such things as religion and other types of belief system, systems of morality, law, patterns of family structures and relationships including marriage and the care of dependents (for instance child-rearing), the ascription of social roles and status including gender roles, and so on. It also refers to common assumptions around such things as food and drink, clothing, music, arts and crafts including the production and use of tools, as well as how people should maintain their existence and contribute to the existence of the society (what is now routinely called 'work' in economically developed societies). It should be clear that in this discussion the meaning of culture is 'anthropological', in the sense of covering the broad spectrum of human life, rather than being used evaluatively to make judgements about particular aspects of those elements just listed such as music and the arts (for example, compare Kuper, 1999, with Jenks, 1993). Another way of saying this would be to note that culture is the overall content of the ways of life of a distinctive society or social group. It has to be noted that this notion is contested within anthropology, sociology and politics (for example, see: Kymlicka, 1989, 1995; Benhabib, 2002, 2004; Eriksen, 2006). However, although these long-standing debates about the validity of this concept can be observed, the notion of culture has greatly influenced the understanding of norms and values that inform consideration of institutions and practices in modern societies. As the following discussion shows, culture must be seen to include social work and human services and the social issues with which they are concerned.

Another way of expressing the approach to culture that needs to be taken in this discussion is found in the notion of 'ethnicity' (which is derived linguistically from the Greek εφνος [ethnos], meaning a nation). An early use of this term, in Barth's (1998 [1969]) analysis of group difference, emphasized how in the modern world cultures are related to nationality. For example, a person understands him or her self as Dutch through the ways that the sets of norms and expectations pertaining to this identity are distinguished from those that characterize being English or French. There is a risk that by looking at identity in this way it can appear to be fixed and/or uniform. So when considering culture as ethnic identity it is important to note both that cultures change over time and also that at any one time there will be differences within as well as between cultures regarding the way in which people understand the expression of those things that constitute a culture (Eriksen, 2006).

Because social work and the human services are concerned with culturally contingent things such as family relationships, the care of children, the care of adults who need assistance in daily life, community well-being and other related issues, culture can be expected to shape their institutions and practices. Yet this has only been explicitly recognized relatively recently, in the 1970s (Borelli, 1975). Kolm appears to disagree, arguing that from the earliest days in the late 1800s, some pioneering social workers had included 'socio-cultural factors' in their thinking, but then continues his analysis to admit that 'despite the manifest concern, the professional literature reveals few signs of real integration' (Kolm, 1978, pp. 3–4). In this respect the 1970s and 1980s marked a watershed of rethinking questions of culture as an aspect of social work and human services theory and practice. In those decades a more critical turn even than that anticipated by Kolm began to connect questions of ethnicity to the issue of 'race', that is the conflation of biological characteristics such as skin colour, eye colour and shape, hair type and so on with culture (see, for example, Solomon, 1976; Coombe & Little, 1986). At the heart of this more critical analysis is a concern with 'racism', which Dominelli (2008, p. 9) defines as 'the politicization of racial attributes', generating the oppression of subordinate groups by those who are dominant. Some forms of racism can be focused on culture rather than physical aspects of 'race', such as concentrating on such things as food and dress as compared to skin colour or facial features. Although there had been challenges to racism in the work of individual practitioners and groups, it was in the late decades of the twentieth century that social work theory can be said to have engaged more thoroughly with this issue and its implications. Moreover, it often sought to do so in the form of what might be called social-political criticism which involved a rethinking of theories, institutions and practices rather than simply adding 'ethnic sensitivity' or 'cultural awareness' to existing ideas and actions (Solomon, 1976; Dominelli, 2002, 2008). This development occurred in the context of wider critical scholarship concerning the way in which ethnicity is a site of discrimination and oppression in the multicultural societies of the modern world (for example, Basu *et al.*, 1978; Centre for Contemporary Cultural Studies, 1982; Gilroy, 1987). These are issues with which social work and human services have to contend, in their own theory, institutions and practices as well as in the wider society, in relation to people of different ethnicities as both service users and as members of the relevant professional and occupational groups (Solomon, 1976; Caulk, 1980; Stubbs, 1985; Coombe & Little, 1986; Hugman, 1991; Dominelli *et al.*, 2001; Dominelli, 2008).

Recognition of the critical importance of culture, ethnicity and 'race' for social work and the human services forces these professional and occupational groups to take a more conscious approach to understanding the multicultural realities of the societies of which they are part. This includes attention to 'racism' in theory and practice as well as to the various claims that can be made about the way in which culture affects attitudes and values. So the concept of culture is complex, with many different aspects that have to be considered in relation to social structures, history and politics; it does not stand alone. Moreover, in so far as culture is regarded as the set of values and attitudes that are related to societies, communities and groups, then it has to be understood as the basis on which people consider what constitutes a good life and how this should be pursued. So for that reason, it is a crucial aspect of any consideration of social work and the human services including, perhaps even especially, the area of professional ethics.

Values

Values have already been defined above as those things that people hold to be important in life, whether these are personal views or are held collectively with others. In the most straightforward terms, values are those things in life that people consider to be important 'for their own sake' (Railton in Hinman, 2008, p. 139). In other words, the goals that values represent do not require any further justification: a value is an end in itself. So, for example, if a person states that they have a goal to maximize their personal income it might be said that they value wealth. However, it would then have to be asked if this was an end in itself or whether it represented a means to achieving some further goal. Two people who both say that they value maximizing personal income might wish to use a larger income in different ways, one to enjoy a very materially comfortable private life and the other to use towards making improvements in the social circumstances of the wider society by providing funding to an organization that seeks to alleviate poverty. Looked at in this way, the values of these two people can be seen as quite different, even though the original, apparently common goal was stated as income maximization. In these cases, that which becomes clear as the 'end in itself' is actually either achieving personal material comfort or benefitting other members of the society who experience poverty.

It has already been implied that values are not only held independently by individual people but are also shared between people in a society. While it is possible that a single person might hold values that are unique to her or him self, it is more likely that these will be shared in some way with others. Indeed, it is extremely hard to hold values that entirely oppose those of everyone else in a society (Bauman, 1994, pp. 10–11). Even where people stand against the prevailing view they tend to draw on other sets of values that also already have a social point of reference. An historical example of this is Gandhi (1869–1948), an Indian lawyer, activist and spiritual leader who in the first half of the twentieth century led campaigns to end the British colonial occupation of India. At times Gandhi was not widely supported by many other people, but his values had their roots in existing legal, political and religious ideas and if other people had not eventually also come to hold these values he would not have achieved the same historical significance in the history of his country (Parekh, 2010). Other examples of people standing up for apparently unpopular values, but who are supported by others with whom they share their commitments, are Aung San Suu Kyi in Myanmar (Burma) and Nelson Mandela in South Africa.

Although it can be concluded from this that values are socially grounded, it also follows that in no society is there a single set of values to which everyone agrees without question. To the contrary, in many societies values are usually the focus of debate and discussion in both public and private life, in political and religious contexts, among family members and friends, within institutions, professions and so on. At the same time there are also usually sufficient common points on which such discussion and debate can take place. That is, there can be expected to be a common stock of broad concepts that are understood as 'ends in themselves' around which agreement and disagreement can be centred. For example, Kekes (1993) suggests that all societies have ideas about the self, intimacy and the social order, such as what sort of killing is acceptable, some notion of what constitutes a 'family' and the extent to which social norms can be challenged. It is the detail of such beliefs and arrangements that distinguish different cultures. Difference within broad cultures is also possible. There is, it might be said, a 'plurality' of differing values in any setting, but these can be held by people without preventing communication occurring or getting in the way of the everyday life of a society. Societies that operate so that differing value positions can be held are known as 'plural'. For Kymlicka (1989), whose work is considered in more detail below and in subsequent chapters, such a society is based on one common or primary value, namely that of being able freely to live what each of us regards as a good life. However, one of Kymlicka's presuppositions, that the basis for understanding what is 'good' and 'bad' is part of a universally shared human condition, in other words is 'transcultural', is contested both generally and within considerations of social work and human services (for example, see: Azmi, 1997; Gray & Fook, 2004; Gasper, 2006). This point lies at the heart of a recognition of value diversity between cultures. If Kymlicka is correct, then establishing a shared value framework for relationships between cultures is possible, but if he is not then the most that could be hoped for would be to find ways of cultures co-existing separately while each pursues its own values.

This is the problem of 'pluralism' and associated questions about the freedom of groups within a society to pursue values that are different and may even be in conflict with each other (Kekes, 1993; Chang, 1997; Hinman, 2008). Hinman (2008) defines pluralism as a third, distinctive position that is different from both absolutism (only one value position can be right) and relativism (all value positions can be seen as right, because any position can only be judged in its own terms). These two opposites often set the terms of debates between value positions; for Hinman, pluralism establishes a third position that is not simply a compromise between the other two. The complexity of pluralism is compounded by Hinman's recognition that there are two forms of relativism: cultural relativism (what is seen as good or right is associated with cultures and the differences between them) and ethical relativism (what is seen as good or right differs relative to the way in which people think about how to decide between possible actions). This concept is examined in depth in Chapter 6. However, at the start of this discussion it is important to identify that it reflects the problem that lies at the centre of the relationship between culture and ethics, namely that in the multicultural situations that exist in very many parts of the world, explicitly identifying and responding to this issue is necessary for any conception of how what is good or right in social work and human services can be examined and understood.

Timms (1983, pp. 2–4) makes the comment that in social work the notion of values is often used but without achieving clarity about which values, whose values they are and to what purpose values might be applied in thinking about institutions and practices. He criticizes social workers and others in the human services for using 'values-talk' to try to associate their work with particular political, religious or other more broadly social values without appearing to recognize that this is what they are doing. It is not that Timms thinks there can be 'value-free' professions, rather that he seeks more explicit attention to the way in which values have to be justified and debated. They cannot simply be used as if they are self-explanatory. What Timms is arguing for is greater effort in developing explanations and justifications for the values that are embedded in social welfare institutions and practices. The challenges to practitioners illustrated in the hypothetical situations with which this chapter began portray the concrete realities faced in the human services.

Ethics

Quite simply, ethics is the 'conscious consideration of our moral values' (Hinman, 2008, p. 5). Recognition of the importance of values being more explicitly addressed in social work and human services has led to a substantial increase in discussions of ethics since Timms (1983) made his criticism about ill-defined 'values-talk' (Shardlow, 1989; Hugman & Smith, 1995; Hugman, 1998, 2005; Congress, 1999; Reamer, 1999; Clark, 2000; Fry & Johnstone, 2002; Banks & Nøhr, 2003, 2011; Beckett & Maynard, 2005; Banks, 2006, 2010; Bowles *et al.*, 2006; Corey *et al.*, 2007; Banks & Gallagher, 2009; Barsky, 2009; Clifford & Burke, 2009; Francis, 2009; Fry *et al.*, 2010; Gray & Webb, 2010; Parrott, 2010; Sercombe, 2010). So, as the centrality of values to theory and practice has become widely recognized, attention to ethics has appropriately followed. Some of the rapidly expanding literature in this field takes the form of 'guides' to practice, that is recommendations and even formulae for the ways in which practitioners can think about ethics in specific situations, while others are wider conceptual discussions about values and principles. However, all in some way explicitly address the question of values, looking not only at the goals of human service institutions and practices but also the connections between such goals and the means used to achieve them.

The predominant approaches to professional ethics in the early twenty-first century are largely derived from the ways of thinking about what is 'good' and what is 'right' that emerged from the processes of modernization that began in Western Europe in the late mediaeval period (Bauman, 1995). As in other areas of life, scientific rationality increasingly displaced tradition, including religion, as the basis for understanding the world and choosing how to act appropriately within it. So moral philosophers began to seek rational principles in the manner of natural science, observing the world and drawing conclusions based on logic in place of rhetoric and revelation. In the development of moral philosophy in Western Europe in this period there are two broad approaches that can be identified: the ethics of duty (what should be done because it is right in itself); and the ethics of consequences (what should be done because it is right in terms of the outcome). These two approaches are known technically as deontology (from the Greek δεον [deon], meaning duty or necessity) and consequentialism. The deontological approach that has been most influential derives from the work of the German philosopher, Kant (1724–1804), whose formulation of principles, which he called 'imperatives', has similarities with the attempts by his contemporaries to discover scientific laws (MacIntyre, 1998; Rachels, 2003). The most influential form of consequentialism has been that of the utilitarians (Bentham [1748–1832] and J. S. Mill [1806–1873]), who sought to apply rational calculation to the balance of outcomes from actions (utility here referring to the usefulness or gain of a particular action) (Rachels, 1998; Hinman, 2008). More recently other ethical approaches have begun to attract (or re-attract) interest, such as virtue ethics and the ethics of care (MacIntyre, 1983; Tronto, 1993) and these will be discussed in subsequent chapters.

The importance of identifying deontology and consequentialism as key to the modern era is in the relationship that they have with the values that have become dominant through this period, values that are expressed in our social and political structures and have effects throughout all aspects of social relationships. Such values include those of individual freedom and of the moral equality of all people. These values can be said to exist in some form in earlier ways of thinking (for example some religions teach that all people should be considered equally as moral beings). However, the modern era is characterized by the translation of the notion of moral freedom and equality into more concrete social arrangements in the relationship between individual people and the wider society (Kymlicka, 1989; Benhabib, 2002; Modood, 2007). The idea of political, economic and social rights and the forms of democracy that are now seen as undeniably 'Western' do not have their origins in traditional Western European cultures but were created in the debates and struggles of recent centuries. These are ideas for which people lost their lives and over which wars and revolutions have been fought. As we will see below, these values are the foundations of the claims by a profession such as social work to be built on principles of human rights and social justice (IFSW/IASSW, 2000/2001, 2004).

A major feature of ethics in the modern, scientific age has been the creation of 'codes of ethics' for professions. Although the ideas that are used to formulate codes are often much older, the concept of a code as an essential part of a profession only emerged in the twentieth century. Prior to that there was a tradition of making moral commitments to serve others with the skills and knowledge derived from a particular training, as in the Hippocratic oath in medicine (Koehn, 1994). However, the development of codes, especially those that are detailed and lengthy, is an expression of the scientific rationalism of the modern era. It was not until the middle of the twentieth century that conventional scholarship and, increasingly, public opinion had come to regard a formal code of ethics as a hallmark of professionalism (Greenwood, 1957; Freidson, 1994). Being able to specify clearly to others what constitutes 'good' practice by members of a profession or occupation thus has come to be seen as a way of guaranteeing openness to those who are not members. Indeed, in recent times codes of ethics often have come to be seen as forming a sort of moral 'contract' with the public and can provide the basis for legal accountability (Koehn, 1994; Reamer, 1999).

Not all analysis of ethics is positive. Bauman (1993, 1994, 1995, 2001a) in particular has argued that a concern with ethics has become a constraint on moral responsibility. This criticism has several aspects. First, he argues that a code of ethics takes away from people their obligation to be consciously engaged with the rightness or wrongness of their actions or of having to think through their values in relation to their relationships with others. Second, Bauman (1993, 1994) points to particular aspects of modern society that use formal ethics as a way of actually limiting moral responsibility: bureaucracy and business. Bureaucracy, he claims, takes away from people the capacity for moral reflection because it reduces human decision making to 'following the correct procedures'; in contrast, business turns all questions of responsibility into matters of contract. Third, in a social world where the dynamics of laws and rules do not compel people to engage with morality but instead limit their capacity to do so, people may often cease to accept that they have any such responsibilities at all (Bauman, 2001a).

However, the defence of ethics in the professions is that it is precisely because people come to the relationship between professionals and service users with a wide range of personal values and beliefs that some sort of formal public statement is necessary (Koehn, 1994; Hugman, 2005; Banks, 2006). Such encounters are the meeting of strangers, at least in so far as the primary focus of the relationship is regarded. Indeed, many professions explicitly identify appropriate role boundaries as an ethical expectation of their members; for example, when providing a service the recipients cannot be treated as if they were friends or family (YACWA, 2003; AASW, 2010). Some may even go so far as to recommend that members do not provide certain sorts of practice for people with whom they already have such a relationship. This position goes against the values of some cultures, where developing such primary relationships in helping is expected (Mafile'o, 2006). (This point will be pursued in later chapters.) Yet, by having a formal code of ethics, service users do not have to negotiate responsibility, trust and so on, each time they encounter a new helper, but can rely on a level of expectation that is provided collectively. This is particularly important as in almost all such situations there is a power imbalance in the relationship. Especially when the helping role also involves some mandated authority, but even simply because professionals possess skills and knowledge that service users may well not do, it is usual for the relationship to be one which all involved experience as unequal. Of course a formal code of ethics does not prevent any individual from acting badly, but it provides a shared basis for considering whether actions are bad or good and also provides for some redress when trust is violated.

It is also the case that many human service organizations have 'standards of practice' or 'codes of conduct' that are independent of any particular profession or occupational group (Webster, 2010). These also have the same overt purpose as codes of ethics, to provide accountability by stating the values of an organization in terms of standards against which actions can be judged. However, for some critics this development raises the possibility of Bauman's concerns about rationalities such as those of business or bureaucracy excluding personal moral responsibility from the relationships between people. In particular, the problem being identified here is that ethics ought to engage everyone in thinking about and taking responsibility for the connections between values and actions (Benhabib, 2002; Hugman, 2005; Banks, 2006; Houston, 2009; Webb, 2009). In contrast, standards of practice or codes of conduct are imposed by employing organizations: they are procedural instructions. Such standards or codes may have the virtue of being objective and explicit, but they are imposed by a third party without the possibility of either of the actors in a situation (service user and practitioner) engaging with their meaning. Codes of ethics may run a similar risk, depending on how they are used, but they are derived from professional or occupational groups in which (at least potentially) each member has both the opportunity and the responsibility to be involved in open discussion to establish and review the values that are expressed. For this reason, codes of ethics are widely supported as the basis for seeing a profession as a moral community, in which each member is called on to be part of the process of dialogue and debate concerning the values that are shared by the members of such a community.

Social work and human services

This book addresses a relatively broad field, that of social work and human services. Professional social work now exists in 87 countries, as recognized by the membership of the International Federation of Social Workers (IFSW), and is developing in several more parts of the world (IFSW, 2011). Yet even among the national bodies representing practitioners who make up the membership of IFSW, all of whom are identified as social workers, there are wide variations in theories and methods of practice, in the focus of their work, in the length and type of education and training required and in whether there is a legal restriction on the title of social worker (Healy, 2008; Hugman, 2010). Working together, the International Association of Schools of Social Work (IASSW) and the IFSW have proposed the following definition of social work.

> The social work profession promotes social change, problem solving in human relationships and the empowerment and liberation of people to enhance well-being. Utilising theories of human behaviour and social systems, social work intervenes at the points where people interact with their environments. Principles of human rights and social justice are fundamental to social work.
>
> (IFSW/IASSW, 2000/2001)

The complexity of this definition and its breadth point to the way in which reaching agreement on the defining characteristics of social work is extremely difficult. As Banks (2006, pp. 2–3) observes, the more detailed a description of social work becomes, the more specific to a particular country it must necessarily be. In some parts of the world there is an emphasis on working with individuals and families, while in others social work focuses on achieving changes in social systems and structures; in many places both are regarded as part of social work (Hugman, 2009). The claims to specific values made in this definition are discussed in more detail in Chapter 2.

It is important to recognize that the theories and practices referred to in the IFSW/IASSW definition have very close parallels with those claimed by other professions or occupations. For example, youth workers, welfare workers and community workers also identify their role as providing assistance to people as individuals, families and communities and as seeking changes in social environments to assist people (Mendes, 2002; YACWA, 2003; Butcher *et al.*, 2007; AIWCW, 2010; Sercombe, 2010). In some counties such roles are regarded as part of social work, in others they are seen as quite distinct although people with formal qualifications in social work also may be employed in positions with these titles (as may practitioners qualified in nursing, occupational theory, psychology, teaching and so on). In yet other countries social work, welfare work and community work may be seen as synonymous and interchangeable terms for a broad service sector that lacks any accepted sense of professionalism.

Similarly, the institutional domains in which these occupations are practised can be distinguished from each other or, in more cases, they are likely to be referred to collectively under generic titles such as social services, social care, community welfare or human services. For example, the term human services is widely used in this way in Australia, Canada and the USA. Interestingly, Banks and her colleagues use the notion of 'the social professions' in order both to identify what such occupations share in their focus and methods and to separate this group from those who are indentified within the concept of 'health professions', such as nurses, occupational therapists, physiotherapists, psychologists and so on (Banks, 2004; Banks & Nøhr, 2003, 2011; Banks & Gallagher, 2009). This construct is clear in that the shared focus of these occupations is the 'social' (as opposed, say, to the biological) aspects of the issues and problems with which people require assistance, as well as to the methods of practice that are used. At the same time, however, this concept remains relatively open and has the same lack of specificity shown by other terms. Other terms include 'people professions' (Bondi *et al.*, 2011) and 'caring professions' (Hugman, 1991, 1998, 2005) and these constructions all include very similar lists of specific professions and occupations. In summary, breadth, interdisciplinarity and a lack of clear boundaries are a feature of this field in most countries, as Banks acknowledges (2006, p. 3).

The inquiry from which this book began has its origins in social work as that is defined by the professional organizations (IFSW/IASSW, 2000/2001). Research and scholarship in this particular occupational area is much more extensive than within either the other distinct professions that might be included under headings, such as 'social', 'people', or 'caring' professions, or the wider human services sector. Medicine, nursing and the allied health professions are obvious exceptions in terms of professions with extensive literatures on ethics, but they are not always included within the concepts of 'social' or 'caring' professions, or as part of the human services. Furthermore, some of the central concerns of this book derive quite explicitly from the international debates that occur in social work. For example, questions of attention to discrimination and oppression in practice as well as in theory have been increasingly addressed in terms of values and ethics in social work for several decades (Solomon, 1976; Coombe & Little, 1986; Langan & Day, 1992; Dominelli, 2002, 2008; Clifford & Burke, 2009). So the focus of the discussion in this book seeks to bring together both social work and the wider field of human services, recognizing that at times this will appear to be emphasizing one over the other. Wherever possible such prioritization will be avoided and it is an underlying supposition of this analysis that much of what is debated in social work is applicable in the wider human services, and *vice versa*, so when the arguments are specific to social work, youth work, community work or any other professional group it is expected that readers will make comparisons and transfer ideas for themselves.

The value terrain of contemporary human services

In order to begin to examine the basis of values in the human services, what can be understood as the value terrain, it is important to bring together the idea of values as those things that are important for their own sake (see above) with an analysis of the type of society that can enable such things to be pursued. It must be remembered that modern social work and human services have developed in an era of industrialized and urbanized societies that are based ideologically on liberalism and rationalism. In the area of knowledge science is the prevailing approach, while in politics such societies are based on principles of democracy. Indeed, some of the early social work pioneers explicitly allied the profession with such ideas (see Addams, 2002 [1907]; also Payne, 2005).

Recognition of this foundation for social work and human services raises important challenges. For example, do the social origins of these professions and services mean that they cannot be developed in countries that do not share all of the characteristics of those where they first emerged? Even within the countries where these professions and services were first created, does this analysis suggest that they are inevitably allied to certain ideas and positions, such as those of particular political parties or of specific religions or ethnicities, and so on? Are there social conditions under which it is unlikely that social work and human services can develop and function, either because they would have no socially accepted purpose or else because the ideas and practices that they embody are seen as an affront to other values and practices?

The international definition of social work, quoted above, is unequivocal in its alliance of the profession with the principles of human rights and social justice. As has also been identified, the ethical statements from other professions and occupations, such as youth work, welfare work and community work, identify the same foundational principles. Yet although recent debates have begun also to focus on questions of culture and ethnicity, especially with regard to the question of racism and other discriminations, relatively little attention has been paid to the underlying questions about the way in which culture, values and, consequently, ethics intersect. These important questions relate not only to understanding the practices and institutions of social work and the human services, but also to considerations of their very existence.

Underlying the assumptions that provide the basis for values and ethics in social work and human services are wider claims about the type of society to which the goals set out by these professions and occupations (social change, problem solving in human relationships, empowerment and liberation for human well-being) are clearly directed. Such societies have been analysed by social, political and economic theorists and philosophers such as Sen (1985, 1999, 2004), Kymlicka (1989, 1995), Nussbaum (1998, 2000, 2006), Benhabib (2002, 2004, 2006) and Modood (2007) as liberal. This term points to the idea of sufficient liberty for individuals to pursue those things that are valued for their own sake as the central principle in all aspects of social structures and relationships.

However, as these theorists all point out, in a multicultural world, especially within multicultural nations, this principle inevitably leads to the 'problem' of pluralism that has been identified above. In summary, this is the challenge of finding ways in which people whose cultural differences lead them to seek divergent ways of living can exist together in the same physical and social spaces. The illustrative practice situations described at the beginning of this chapter show that such questions are not only important at the level of broad theory or policy but also in day-to-day practice. How social workers and other human services practitioners comprehend the relationship between culture, values and ethics and incorporate this understanding in their work will affect their responses to the people for whom they seek to provide a service. The decisions faced by Julie, Farouk and Alan about expressions of culture, the position of girls and young women in their service, and so on, are central to their work. Similarly, Imelda's responses to Gunawathie and her family are not simply about whether she has grasped facts about a culture different to her own and so become more 'ethnically competent', but that she is also explicitly aware of the way in which her practice affects the human agency of each person who is involved. In both situations, the wider value of freedom to make choices about what is important for its own sake in life is central to decisions about wearing *hijab*, having separate gender-based services or disclosing bad news about someone's health status. Yet, in both situations, the question remains that each choice for decision and action may be questioned from cultural standpoints in which it is not accepted that the basic premise of freedom to make choices about what matters is a property of individuals. It is this challenge that is faced by social work and human services and which this book addresses.

The structure and overall argument of this book

This chapter has identified the interconnected issues of culture, values and ethics for social work and the human services. The discussion here provides an introduction to the themes that are developed in the following chapters. There are five core questions arising from these themes.

- First, how do issues of culture affect the ways in which social work and human services grasp and respond to the relationship between values and ethics?
- Second, following from this, why is it important to consider culture and cultural values when considering professional values and ethics?

- Third, in what ways do the practices and institutions of social work and human services relate to the aspirations people have of the good society and the right way to live?
- Fourth, how can social work and human services grasp and respond to the reasonable differences that people might have about the values that are expressed by such aspirations?
- Fifth, how will answering these questions assist social work and human services in the future development of 'good' practice?

In order to answer these questions, the book examines critical aspects of culture, values, ethics and the professions. In Chapter 2 the implications of culture for social work and human services practices are considered in greater depth. In particular, the chapter explores further the inherently cultural nature of many of the social and interpersonal problems and challenges in response to which these practices and institutions have developed. It also looks at the ways in which the understanding of these issues differs between countries, presenting particular problems for international relationships within the professions concerned. Chapter 3 then focuses on the professions and the importance of ethics as part of professionalism. It makes connections between the question of value differences for international relationships and for thinking about multicultural dialogue and exchanges about these matters.

Chapters 4 and 5 in turn examine the competing claims of universalism and cultural relativism in considerations of values and ethics. The former argues that in order to think about professional practice and service provision in modern, multicultural societies it is necessary to begin from an understanding of shared humanity. In other words, the foundations of professional values and ethics should be a vision of what it is to be human that does not depend on context or other contingencies. In particular, human rights and social justice depend on this approach, because they make such claims. Cultural relativism, on the other side of the argument, places great emphasis on the particularities of the ways in which different people have different ideas about those things that matter for their own sake in life and that these are formed in particular cultures. Chapter 6 then moves into the area of ethical pluralism, to consider the way in which the recognition of difference does not necessarily require the abandonment of shared values or of the possibility of dialogue and agreement between cultural positions. This discussion also introduces some of the more recent approaches in ethics, especially those that are grounded in thinking about social relationships and communication.

In Chapter 7 the area of spirituality and religion is considered as a particular expression of cultural values. This is an aspect of social life that has not always been addressed by social work and human services theory. Its significance for thinking about multicultural practice is a major theme of the chapter. Then Chapters 8 and 9 address particular theoretical issues raised by the preceding discussion. The first of these is ethical pluralism and its relationship to particular ideas about politics and social structures. In other words, do modern social work and human services depend on certain forms of democracy in order to be able to function? This debate has significance again for the claims to human rights and social justice as foundational principles. The second problematic issue, examined in Chapter 9, is that of the 'paradox' of value differences that can be seen in the counter claims between (1) notions of individual freedom to choose values and (2) the assertion of the rights of cultural communities to establish the choices available to their members. In conclusion, Chapter 10 examines ways in which social work and human services can embrace diversity, by looking at the possible relationship between notions of shared humanity and cultural difference.

Overall, this is a book about the nature and scope of contemporary social work and human services. It is written from the perspective that it is vital in a multicultural world, in which everyone has rights, most especially to our identities and our values, that professions and services can help to sustain and extend human capabilities to achieve those things that we each see as important for their own sake in life.

2 The implications of culture for social work and human services

Introduction

Social work and all other areas of the human services are inherently value laden. The core professional concerns focus on aspects of life about which people hold very strong values and opinions. These include child-rearing and child-care; the development of children and young people; other aspects of family relationships including those between partners or couples; the social care of people with health problems including both physical and mental health; support for those people with disabilities who need assistance; the social dimensions of problems faced by older people; and issues and challenges faced by specific groups within the community, such as refugees, as well as wider questions concerning the development of policies and institutions that address these various aspects of personal and social life. Professions such as social work have also played an important role in the definition of social needs and the creation of policies and practices that address these (Addams, 2002 [1907]; Payne, 2005). In many parts of the world the various ways in which social work has developed as a profession is also a reflection of the structural (macro-level) understanding of social well-being, such that social development and community work are also regarded as important areas of practice, alongside the more intrapersonal and interpersonal focus of counselling, casework, couple and family therapy, social service administration and so on (Hugman, 2009). In other places social development and community work are considered as separate professional fields (Butcher *et al.*, 2007).

These are all aspects of people's lives about which there are different and often competing ideas. That is, it is not only possible but entirely reasonable that such ideas will be discussed, debated and contested within as well as between different cultural contexts. There are three particular implications of this for social work and the human services that are central to this analysis. The first is that there are competing understandings about the goals of social welfare and human services: what are they there to achieve? Why are they provided? Should they be provided professionally; or should they be provided at all? Second, there is often disagreement about the policies and institutions that are appropriate for the provision of social welfare services (O'Connor *et al.*, 2006; Lymbery, 2007). Should such services be provided by government or by independent agencies? Who should be involved in forming policies and how should that process occur? Should professionals influence policy or should they be directed by others? How should the work of professionals and others be directed and managed? Third, the very practices of social work and human services are open to similar sorts of value-laden debate. The core question here is that of *who* should determine how these service providers should act. In this respect we may say that social workers and human services providers face a degree of scrutiny similar to that often experienced in school teaching, nursing and other areas in which the degree to which claims over professional knowledge and skills are less exclusive than in some of the 'classic' professions (Hugman, 1991). In other words, these are practices that depend on the specialized application of what can appear to be everyday social skills and ideas. Yet these practices occur within contexts where there are also discrete levels of skill and knowledge that may be unknown to those without relevant training and which are not necessarily recognized or accepted as specialized because of strong cultural values about what is 'right' and 'good'. Examples of areas in which expertise is not necessarily acknowledged can be seen in arguments about 'what should be done about/with/for young people who commit crimes' or 'how and by whom should care services for older people be provided'.

In order to examine these issues in more depth, this chapter explores them at three different levels. To begin, it asks what are the concerns of social work and the human services, considered broadly, and how do they relate to cultural values. To do this it takes specific examples and considers them in depth. Then, the discussion narrows a little to examine the challenges posed internationally by the variation between cultures concerning values around the core concerns. Finally, the chapter looks at how questions of cultural values relate to the international definition of social work (IFSW/IASSW, 2000/2001) and the implications this has not only for the issues that have been considered so far but also for the boundaries between social work and other professions and occupations in human services. This final question establishes a connection with significant debates about professionalism that are then explored in Chapter 3.

Cultural values in social work and human services practice

In broad terms, we can consider the central concern of social work and the human services as the promotion of human well-being within the social context. Indeed, this is reflected in the long-standing way of describing social work, in order to distinguish its orientation from those of other professions, as a focus on 'the person within their social environment', which some commentators regard as the foundation of social work's concern with the value of social justice (Lundy, 2004; Figueira-McDonough, 2007, pp. 188–189; Green & McDermott, 2010). In other words, social work seeks to promote change both for individual people and for the social structures within which people live their lives. However, as will be discussed in more detail below, this distinction can also lead to clear positions developing both inside and outside social work that seek to prioritize one or the other (Hugman, 2009). As we will see, giving different weight to the individual and to the societal levels of understanding human need can at times represent national, if not cultural, sets of values (especially political values, which as we saw in Chapter 1 are closely interconnected with ethics). This occurs because the definition of well-being itself is inevitably constructed from the notions of 'good' and 'right' that are very much part of every culture. Thus it has to be acknowledged at the outset that the core focus of the social welfare field is itself comprised of values and that these differ between cultures.

The first concrete example of practice, policy and service provision that will be examined is that of child welfare. This area of human life can be said to be one of the most important in the values of all cultures (Jenks, 1996; Baxter, 2005). In common with all living organisms human beings must reproduce in order to continue the exist-ence of the species. Indeed, since this fact has been recognized throughout history such a statement may appear to be so obvious as to be unnecessary. In a field such as social development, the reduction of infant mortality is regarded as one of the central indicators of a society progressing (Ferrarini & Sjöberg, 2010; Jorgensen & Rice, 2010). Prior to the twentieth century in all countries, and still in many less highly developed nations, children also have often been seen as a resource for the family, the wealth of the future in terms of productive labour, care for family members in their old age and so on. The way in which this basic fact is changed through economic growth and social development, so that in advanced industrial societies children may be seen differently, does not appear to have taken away the sense that children 'belong' to the family (which may be wider than just the biological parents) (Howe, 2005). However, one of the ways in which children are valued that is shared by both developing and highly developed countries is that children are regarded as the future citizens, that is as the literal future of a society. In that sense they may also represent a future 'resource', at least at the collective level in the case of the economically most highly developed societies (Jenks, 1996).

At an individual level attention must also be given to the psychological attachment that parents usually have towards their children (Howe *et al.*, 1999; Howe, 2005). A central concern of social work and human services in many countries is when these attachments are not developed or are disrupted in some way, so that children are neglected or maltreated. While there are widely differing cultural norms about what constitutes 'good' treatment of children, there is no evidence of any culture system-atically approving a disregard for the well-being of children (Jenks, 1996; Baxter, 2005). So, it might be expected that in all cultures there is some concept of what is acceptable and what is not in relation to the appropriate care of a child, even though in detail there will be differences between cultures. Thus, the exact definition of child neglect and maltreatment might be expected to vary in detail between different coun-tries. For example, in relation to the cultural forms that the expression of care might take, people in all of these situations can be expected to share a sense that young children are vulnerable and require nurturing (Baxter, 2005; Parton, 2009). In each situation, therefore, there are expectations about what should be done by parents and other family members, neighbours and the wider community and the society as a whole. So the ethics of child-care and child-rearing, while having a shared foundation across all human societies, is embedded in cultural norms in its concrete expression in everyday life. Where this becomes an ethical challenge is when different cultures encounter each other and child-care and child-rearing practices become open to scrutiny from different positions. In particular, there are questions of the power of professionals who tend to have their cultural and ethical points of reference in dominant social positions, whether these are derived from differences of 'race' and ethnicity, socio-economic class or an interweaving of the two (Dominelli, 2008). This can occur both when people from one cultural background migrate to another country and also in the practice of social welfare professionals in international non-government organizations (INGOs) such as Save the Children, UNICEF and the International Committee of the Red Cross (Healy, 2008; Hugman, 2010).

To illustrate this complex point, let us consider the following hypothetical situation.

> Vumani Botshoma is a four year old boy whose family have migrated from Botswana to Australia. Vumani's father is a mining technician and has a highly paid job. The Botshoma family live in a major city while Mr Botshoma works many hundreds of kilometres away, flying to and from his work so he is away for many days and then at home for similar periods of time. Vumani is attending a pre-school group run by the local Migrant Resource Centre, where the teacher, Pauline, notices that he often comes to the group with bruising on his legs and his arms. Pauline is aware that there are also two older children, girls aged 6 and 9, attending a local state primary school; she is also aware that Mrs Botshoma has spoken with other staff at the Centre about finding life in Australia difficult and often feeling isolated when her husband is away. Recognizing that there may be a variety of explanations for Vumani's bruises, Pauline expresses concern to Mrs Botshoma and suggests that if it is a case of him bruising easily then maybe Vumani needs to see the health worker who comes to the Centre each week. On learning that Vumani often has to be chastised for bad behaviour and this sometimes involves physical restraint, Pauline tries to explain that under Australian law that physical discipline of children cannot be used when it causes injury. Mrs Botshoma responds by accusing Pauline of judging her because she is an ethnic minority migrant and of not understanding 'African values'; she then withdraws Vumani from the pre-school group. Because of the laws that apply to suspected mistreatment of a child, Pauline then communicates her concerns to the government welfare agency that is mandated to investigate suspicions of child maltreatment and the case is allocated to a social worker, Lauren. When Lauren visits the family she is met by both Mr and Mrs Botshoma who are very angry and who accuse Lauren, the agency and the wider community of racism, of trying to stop them from bringing up their children well within their cultural norms and of failing to support families who come from other countries when they face difficulties in settling in a new country. After a long argument they eventually agree to try to change how they discipline Vumani and to accept Lauren visiting to monitor the situation, but 'only because of the legal implications'.

Although the details of this situation are hypothetical, in broad terms it matches the experiences of migrants and of social welfare professionals in many advanced industrial countries, where clashes between people's understanding of their own cultural values and those of a new country can often be encountered (see, for example: McMahon, 2005; Chang *et al.*, 2006; Healy, 2007). (It should also be noted that this example is not used to single out African migrants to Western countries as 'inadequate parents' [see: Robinson, 2007; Dominelli, 2008]. Such differences and disagreements with law, policy and practice may be encountered with people from many backgrounds, including families among the cultural majority community [see: Roberts, 2000; Whitney *et al.*, 2006].)

The example of the Botshoma family raises several ethical issues, including questions of rights, agency, autonomy, freedom, care and responsibility. These include both the actions of individuals and also the structural relationships between groups of people as professionals and service users, migrants and members of a majority culture, children and adults, and so on. At the centre of the situation is the question of whether parents have the right to discipline their children using whatever means seem to them to be appropriate. There is no doubt that there are broad cultural values shared between Australia and Botswana that good parents will exercise discipline over their children, ensure that children learn to act well within the society and so grow up well and avoid conflict with others. The challenge in this instance is that the predominant view of the use of physical chastisement in Australian and other Western societies is that it not only harms children physically, especially when it causes injury, but also that it causes psychological and moral harm (Roberts, 2000; Gershoff, 2002). The latter aspect concerns the way in which such means of discipline undermines the integrity of the child's person (their body and their developing sense of self) and so limits their human agency even when this is understood in age-appropriate terms. This view is embodied in the United Nations' *Convention on the Rights of the Child* (CRC) (UN, 1989). However, there are ethnicities, including cultural subgroups in Western countries, in which it remains normative to use physical chastisement in meeting the goal of disciplining children (Roberts, 2000; Gershoff, 2002; Rhee, 2003; Chang *et al.*, 2006; Ibanez *et al.*, 2006; Whitney *et al.*, 2006). Consequently the CRC and other international conventions and instruments are criticized from some perspectives as the imposition of Western values on non-Western cultures, or of dominant perspectives on cultural minorities.

Alongside this point, we must also consider the rights of parents, which within both Western and African cultural values are widely considered as primary (that is, as an important, general and overarching value, see discussion in Chapter 1). From a pluralistic and multicultural view of ethics it is reasonable to expect that the detail of particular expressions of such a value will differ between contexts. That is, the specific form that the exercise of parental rights takes, such as the use of physical chastisement, should be considered as a secondary value. So it can be agreed that in neither cultural context are parents accorded total freedom in how they might choose to exercise their responsibilities in any aspect of parenting. In both settings there are debates and differences of opinion about such values. For example, in relation to the illustrative case above, some mainstream Australians (those of European descent) may also challenge the prevailing views about limitations on how parents discipline their children and be equally angry at the intervention of social workers or other professionals (Roberts, 2000).

It is also the case that professionals working in the field of child-care and child protection may differ between Western countries in the detail and the orientation of their values. While the broad aspects as already described may be shared, there can be national differences. For example, Hort (1997) has argued that social workers in Sweden tend to regard the cultures of migrant families as contributory to child welfare problems and see their role as including cultural education. Christie (2010) makes a similar point about Ireland, arguing that the country's child welfare policies and practices reinforce 'white Irish' cultural norms. Kriz and Skivenes (2010) compared Norway and England and found that while in the former cultural diversity is valued, in the latter there is an emphasis on balancing cultural sensitivity with a concern for children's safety; again, the dominant ethnic understanding of such issues is the implicit norm. These findings are supported by Williams and Soydan (2005) in a comparison of Sweden and the UK. So although such variations may appear to be subtle, between these Western European countries there are different ways of understanding and acting on what in broader terms is a shared cultural assumption about the values of 'good' parenting.

From these arguments it may be understood that professionals such as Pauline and Lauren in the illustrative case example above are not simply working on the basis of their own values or their personal interpretation of their professions' ethics. While these have a significance for how they act as individuals in relation to other individuals, both the ethical codes of their professions and the laws and policies that mandate their practices in this particular country place quite specific requirements on them in their roles as a teacher and a social worker. In this situation the paramount concern is understood as that of the safety and well-being of children. This in turn is perceived in terms of the child's rights to care and freedom from harm, which over-ride certain rights of others and place obligations on those others (parents, professionals, the wider society) to act in certain ways. In the language of human rights, the child is the rights holder and the responsible adults are the duty bearers (O'Neill, 2005). Thus the rights of children limit the rights of adults in quite specific ways in defined circumstances. But from a perspective that understands the accountability of parents as belonging to their wider family, to elders within the wider community, to religious leaders, or to a combination of these, the actions of professionals under the authority of the state can be experienced as an affront to deeply held values and so as a criticism of their cultural identity (Azmi, 1997; Rhee *et al.*, 2004; Chang *et al.*, 2006). This is so, irrespective of whether the use of physical chastisement, or degree of its use, is regarded as appropriate or otherwise.

A similar extent of cultural differences can be observed in the care of older people. Here again there is a clear variation between the Western cultures that predominate in the advanced industrial countries and those in all other parts of the world. In Western societies, over several centuries, the normative expectations that those older people who need care and assistance will be looked after by their offspring or other family members have gradually been modified to the extent that by the end of the twentieth century it has become much more common for families to seek professional care for older members who require such assistance and for social policy to support this with both at-home and out-of-home services often supported, either in whole or partly, through tax-based funding (at least in some countries). The following brief (hypothetical) example from an assessment team for services for older people illustrates this issue.

Shu-Mei is a community nurse; born and raised in Singapore in the Chinese community, she migrated to Australia as a young adult where she trained and has since practised. Geoff is a social worker; his family migrated to Australia several generations ago, mostly from the UK but also from Ireland and The Netherlands. He trained in Australia and has also worked for two years in the UK. They are colleagues in a state government Department of Health 'aged-care assessment team'. Shu-Mei and Geoff are involved in the assessment of Jean Robinson, aged 82, who lives on her own with some support from family members who live in another part of the same city, especially her daughter Jill who is aged 53. Mrs Robinson is now severely disabled, both physically and mentally, and the family members are finding it increasingly difficult to provide the necessary level of care, so they have requested an assessment for a place in a nursing home. This is particularly affected by the fact that it takes her daughter almost an hour travelling to visit her mother and in addition she has recently been offered a more senior position at work which she is keen to take both for the role in itself and because the additional salary will assist in supporting her own daughter who has recently started at university. Mrs Robinson is not keen to leave the home where she has lived for over 40 years but the family are insistent that they cannot now cope with all that providing care requires. Jill feels ambivalent about this and expresses distress about 'letting her mother down' but at the same time also feels strong obligations to her husband and children. In discussing the situation, Shu-Mei and Geoff agree that their priorities are to focus on the needs of Jean Robinson and also of Jill, which in this case should be regarded as at a high level. However, in their discussion it is clear that Shu-Mei is more sympathetic to Jill's ambivalence and her feeling of obligation to her mother while Geoff places more weight on the idea that Jean Robinson's moral claims on her daughter are limited by Jill's choice to prioritize the needs and interests of her daughter and husband as well as her own needs and interests such as in her career options. Shu-Mei and Geoff conclude that it is helpful that they can reach agreement by focusing on the mandate of their agency role so that they do not have to reach their recommendation on the basis of their different value perspectives. They also agree that Mrs Robinson's wishes to remain in her own home are very important: the question is whether this can be facilitated without the family's continuing high level of direct care.

This example shows a difference in value perspectives brought to bear in the situation, but also indicates that these can be subtle and have to be understood in context.

This illustration portrays a common set of circumstances in a Western country, one that is also increasingly common in other parts of the world, especially those Asian countries that are economically highly developed or developing rapidly. Although the Western model of social security and professionalized care for older people has been critiqued frequently from Asian and African perspectives (Koyano, 2000; Kaseke, 2005), the scale of cultural difference in values between different parts of the world can be questioned and also whether values within any culture ought to be regarded as unitary. For example, Spira and Wall (2009) note that in many modernizing societies the demands of traditional culture may need to be modified to accommodate to the realities faced by younger family members in employment.

First, it is more plausible to see the Western pattern of such arrangements as a response to rapid shifts in the demographics and economies of advanced industrial countries. Quite simply, in circumstances where it is now common for all members of a household to be in employment or education, previous patterns of there being family members (usually women) available to care for older relatives cannot continue to operate as they had done in previous eras (Finch, 1989). It is the changes in social structures and other social relationships (gender relations, patterns of employment and so on) that create the dynamic for such developments, not simply a decline in a sense of obligation to care for older relatives. Indeed, the same pressures are being encountered in Asian countries, such as China and Japan, where professionalized services of the same kind as those found in Western countries have developed (Koyano, 2000; Mjelde-Mossey *et al.*, 2005; Glass *et al.*, 2010). Among Chinese, Japanese and Korean families, it is argued, the need for professionalized services coexists uncomfortably with the Asian value of filial piety (the responsibility of children, especially sons, to honour their parents) (Koyano, 2000; Asai & Kameoka, 2005; Mjelde-Mossey *et al.*, 2005; Glass *et al.*, 2010).

At the same time, that such changes are experienced in China, Japan and other Asian countries as undermining core values can be said to be matched by the sense in Western countries that professional care, especially out-of-home care such as a nursing home, is the choice of last resort for most people (compare Mjelde-Mossey *et al.*, 2005, with Allen *et al.*, 1992). This can be even more pronounced for migrant families (Spira & Wall, 2009) and the assumption of the value of filial piety is increasingly criticized as a questionable stereotype (Koyano, 2000; Asai & Kameoka, 2005). Western families along with those from other parts of the world continue to feel a sense of moral obligation to provide such care, even if at times this involves giving up what would now widely be regarded as reasonable claims to other valued aspects of life (Finch, 1989; Hughes & Heycox, 2010). That some Asian countries such as Singapore have taken a somewhat different approach and legislated to reinforce the obligations of families actually highlights the pressures felt by many people in the modern economy, in that it suggests that otherwise there might be arguments for the state to take a more active role and to assume responsibility for care arrangements (Mehta, 2006). (At the time of writing China is also considering such legislation.)

It should also be remembered that Western cultures are plural, both in the sense of there being differences between different countries but also between groups and individuals within countries. In broad terms there remains a distinction of values regarding the care of older family members, at least of degree, between the North and the South of Europe, paralleled in those countries that derive their predominant culture from them (in North and South America, and Australasia). But here also, as with Japan, the main factor is how recently the economy has modernized. Where this has been rapid and recent there is a tension between cultural values of family responsibility for care for older members and the economic reality of employment patterns for women. In this respect it is critical to note that assumptions about women performing these caring tasks run across many cultures, whether African, Asian or Western. The challenge to such values therefore can be seen as directly linked to the changes in women's lives through the impact of economic development, education and other aspects of social development.

Similarly, Lum (2005, p. 9) notes that in the USA there is a strong correlation between the ethnicity of families and their economic circumstances, so that care for older African-Americans is more likely to be provided by family members because they are more likely to lack resources to access professional aged care and are also more likely to be part of extended families where people have less secure employment. Yet African-Americans are also the group with the largest proportion of older people without family caregivers, while Hispanic-Americans have the 'most resourceful caregiving networks' but are the most likely to receive care from formal services (p. 17). In this way socio-economic class factors can also be masked by attention to ethnicity and culture; gender has an influence across the ethnic groupings, with women almost twice as likely as men not to receive care, but when they did for that care to be formal services. At the same time Lum cautions that after controlling for such factors there is still a clear impact of cultural values, so this suggests that the different factors must be understood as intersecting and not as determined by one or the other. While the study can be seen as tending to take actual care arrangements (what people do) as representational of cultural values (what people think *should* be done), it demonstrates the way in which culture cannot be separated from other factors. A study by Chow *et al.* (2010) adds to this, noting that Asian and Pacific Islander Americans were also highly unlikely to use formal care services, but here the common explanatory factor is cultural, with socio-economic and other factors differing widely between and within these groups.

Cultural difference and the international definition of social work

From this sketch of some practical aspects of differences in cultural values, using two fields of practice in child welfare and services for older people, the discussion may now be broadened to examine the way in which social work and related areas of human services are defined internationally. As noted in Chapter 1, the way in which social work is constructed as a profession differs between countries, as does the relationship that it has with the wider field of human services including other 'social professions' (Banks, 2004; Lonne *et al.*, 2004). There is a general level of agreement between more than 80 countries about how this field should be defined, although at the more detailed level difference and debate becomes more apparent (Hugman, 2010).

To explain this broad agreement and accompanying debates it is necessary to look again in detail at the 'international definition of social work' as agreed by the International Federation of Social Workers (IFSW) and the International Association of Schools of Social Work (IASSW) (see Chapter 1). In this definition these organizations state that social work 'promotes social change', helps to solve problems 'in human relationships' and seeks to promote 'the empowerment and liberation of people' in order 'to enhance well-being'. This is a very complex understanding, because it was aiming to bring together those countries in which the profession of social work is seen predominantly as providing clinical services and administering social welfare programmes, those where it is overwhelmingly regarded as the agent of structural change and engaged in community practice, including social development, and those in which some balance between the two can be found. For example, in South America a strong emphasis is placed on effecting change in social systems and policies, and valuing 'empowerment' and 'liberation' at the collective level (Elliott & Segal, 2008, p. 352). This contrasts with North America where the predominant way in which social work is practised is in work with individuals and families, so that 'empowerment' and 'liberation' are acknowledged, if at all, through personal problem solving and a focus on human behaviour (Olson, 2007). In both instances, these are trends and do not define all social work and human services practice (Healy, 2008).

The tendency, by some contributors to the debate between micro- and macro-level practice, to over-emphasize one or the other may lead to a distortion of the breadth that makes up social work as a whole and links it with the wider human services (Hugman, 2009). Nevertheless, even when considered as possessing a unifying core, these debates are important for the way in which they also relate to differences in professional values and ethics, and the relationship between those two things. For example, in those contexts in which social work is defined in terms of the promotion of social change and a related focus on social systems as the object of change, the primary values (as stated in the definition) tend to be seen in these terms. That is, human rights are understood in relation to the way that various sectors of a society are advantaged or disadvantaged, whether relatively or absolutely: in other words rights issues are embedded in questions of social justice (Reisch, 2008). Moreover, social justice is understood through an analysis of the way in which resources (whether material or social) are distributed in a society (Reisch, 2002). So, for example, concern might be given to identifying those people who are impoverished as a means of allocating professional attention, access to services and so on. In ethical terms this approach to defining the field rests firmly on utilitarian ideas. It seeks to set priorities between people in terms of social characteristics and thus gives preference to the needs of particular sections of the society. In other words, to achieve the 'greatest good of the greatest number' of people, in this construction of social work and human services, the goal is to direct attention to where it will do most good and to leave those who can access other means for resolving problems to do so. At the same time, it also takes a stand on the origins of social problems, seeing these as lying in social structures that are held to be the cause of disadvantage. From this perspective, attending to human behaviour should only take the form of supporting people to be more effective in their struggles against disadvantage, otherwise it becomes 'victim blaming' (Banks, 2006, p. 38). Attention to human rights therefore follows from social justice: it is seen in terms of emphasizing concern with the lack of access to achieving rights for those who are disadvantaged.

In contrast, the other side of this binary understanding of the field places great emphasis on human rights as a property of each individual person. As Ife (2008) argues, a focus on human rights as political and economic rights limits the potential for seeing rights as belonging to groups or communities. It is this very factor that tends to support arguments that human rights are a Western construct, given the development of individualism and liberalism in European societies over a long period of time. Even defenders of the concept of the right to express a culture and to live within its requirements, such as Kymlicka (1995), nevertheless make it very clear that at no time should the claims of a culture over-ride the right of each person to define and pursue their own concept of 'good' and 'right' (also see Ebadi in UNDP, 2004, p. 23). When applied within social work and the human services, as in the underlying ethos that applies to arguments for the rights of children not to be physically disciplined or the rights of both an older person and her or his family members, such a value is based on the prevailing concept that rights are properties of persons – that is, rights apply to individual people each considered separately, even if in relationship. In ethical terms, this is an approach based on moral duty, in the sense that what is 'right' is considered from the perspective that what applies to one person must be equally available to all, without exception. Therefore each person has a moral duty to respect the humanity of all other people by acting in such a way as to uphold their rights. From this point of view, attention to social justice follows from human rights: it constructs differences, including disadvantage, as contingencies that are a secondary concern and are important because they affect achievement of human rights (which are universal and come before concerns with social justice).

For social work and human services this means that the meaning and significance of human rights may appear very hard to grasp firmly when looked at between cultures and between different positions within cultures. Yet, as Ife (2008, p. 69) along with others (see, for example: Lundy, 2006; Healy, 2008) has pointed out, this denies both the way in which other ideas of human rights are considered and addressed from within non-Western cultures as well as from other Western perspectives. For example, there are many faith traditions and social philosophies that express ideas about human rights even when they do not actually use the specific term (for example, see: Keown, 2007; Sanyal, 2010). The same traditions also have concepts of social justice, in the sense of defining norms about what is fair and reasonable about the distribution of material and social resources; some do so to the extent of arguing that those who are disadvantaged have claims to the assistance of the wider society. So, for this point of view, arguments based on human rights or social justice cannot simply be taken as 'Western'. Cross-cultural issues lie elsewhere, in the definition of what these values mean in practice, who should be able to assert what sort of moral claims, and so on. We will return to this point in later parts of this book.

It also may very well be that social work and human services are challenged by the way in which the human rights of individuals in any given situation can be in conflict, or that contrary claims to what would be just in a given situation are not easily disentangled, and that this is inevitable because some individual needs and interests are different. This is evident in the two hypothetical case situations above. Moreover, the sense of conflict between values can itself be felt by the people involved in these situations themselves. People in many different cultures may want to have their own position recognized and at the same time to act 'well' as a member of a family or a community. This is seen in the instance of Mrs Robinson's daughter Jill in the example outlined above, who has strongly held values of what it is to be a good daughter and a good partner and mother, but finds that what is necessary in order to achieve these values is quite contradictory: she cannot actually accomplish all of them. The professionals who are assessing her mother's needs for care services therefore have to work with this contradiction. For the Botshoma family, the contradiction is between learning to live in a new country while at the same time experiencing this as undermining their strongly held values about good parenting. In this situation the contradiction comes more from external pressures: they would be subject to scrutiny if they were failing to exercise any discipline over their children but at the same time the way that discipline is exercised has to conform to particular values (compare with Christie, 2010). So the situations of both Mrs Robinson and the Botshoma family are perceived as ethically complex by the professionals who are involved with them.

For Baldry (2010) the sense of tension between human rights and social justice as core values for social work and the human services is more apparent than actual. Although the relationship between these two values requires careful thought, for Baldry it can be explained as an interaction between the two. First, human rights are concerned with access to those things that are necessary to live a truly human life. (This point is examined in greater depth in Chapter 4.) Second, social justice is concerned with the way that we distribute social and material resources to meet human needs in a finite world. So the relationship between the two is that human rights are effectively 'what' social justice seeks to have distributed fairly and equitably. That is, the basic question of social justice is why some people are denied human rights, which may take the form of access to material resources, and what can be done to redress this. In turn, social justice grounds human rights in the realities of a finite world. It is not reasonable to expect that in all circumstances achieving the rights of all people will be easy or unproblematic: resources may be limited; the interests of individual people and of groups may be in competition, even contradictory; values that are held individually or collectively may even at times be impossible to reconcile in a given situation (see more detailed discussion in Chapter 9). Some basis must be found for addressing these challenges, both in the day-to-day practice of work by professionals and other service providers, and in the ways in which professions, organizations, governments and wider societies think about the priorities for social policy and human services more generally.

The illustrative hypothetical examples of the Botshoma family and Mrs Robinson's family above embody a range of values and ethical principles. At the broadest they demonstrate issues concerning human rights and social justice. For example, these situations reveal questions of the rights of children with regard to how they are treated by adults, the rights of adults with dependency needs to have those needs considered by others and the rights of adults who have caring responsibilities to be able to balance these with other demands placed on them. They also demonstrate the way that questions of social justice relate to social factors such as age, gender, 'race' and ethnicity and so on. In particular, the issue of social power, that is of who has the socially constructed capacity to make choices and to obtain the co-operation of others, is seen as a question of social justice. For example, would the compliance of the Botshoma family be less easy to obtain if they were 'local' and of greater socio-economic status? Does Jill have a brother and if so does he feel the same ambivalence about providing direct care for Mrs Robinson? These are also questions that will be seen to have diverse meanings in diverse cultural contexts, so that social workers and others in human services in different countries may be expected to put the values of human rights and social justice into practice in ways that appear to be expressing them in very different ways. So the way in which the questions themselves are asked as well as the answers that might follow could be expected to vary between countries.

Cultural difference, values and ethics

From a Western perspective some of the more detailed ways in which values such as human rights and social justice relate to human services practices may appear to be self-evident. As noted above, the discourse of child abuse is now effectively taken for granted – indeed, nothing in the discussion here is intended to imply that harming a child is acceptable: the point is to understand what counts as harm. Other aspects require more specific ethical consideration. For instance, are there limitations concerning who professionals can inform about their concerns regarding possible child maltreatment? How can workers show respect to parents at the same time as investigating possible maltreatment (possibly against the parents' own wishes)? How can careful consideration of each point of view be ensured in an assessment process for an older person's needs? And in relation to both these examples, how should a human services professional deal with any possible dissonance between the values expressed in social policy and requirements of an agency on the one side and their own values on the other? To make sense of broad ideas such as human rights and social justice in concrete situations more specific principles are required. In everyday practice it is more likely that human services professionals will recognize that they pay attention to ethical principles such as privacy and confidentiality, human agency and dignity, care and respect, trust, honesty and so on (Banks, 2004, 2006; Bowles *et al.*, 2006; Congress & McAuliffe, 2006). Yet even these principles, their meaning and how they might be recognized in action, can be understood differently from diverse perspectives. Expressing care and respect, for example, might be demonstrated in one context by giving very direct advice, even instruction, to a service user while in another context this same response might be construed as domination and oppression because respect would be understood in terms of giving the service user a lot of scope to make their own choices.

Nimmagadda and Cowger (1999, pp. 267–268) argue that in a traditional Hindu setting Indian service users would expect the former response from a 'good' practitioner: practitioners 'justified giving advice for three reasons; one, it was their duty; two, it was expected by clients and their families; and three, it works'. In contrast, in a Western context the concept of 'self-determination' is widely regarded as most appropriate (compare with Bowles *et al.*, 2006, pp. 140–143). Interestingly, Yip's (2004) description of Chinese service users' responses to social workers shows that in yet another cultural setting following direct advice or instruction can depend on whether it is the 'right' advice (that is, if it matches other aspects of traditional values, in this case Confucian) and the authority of the professional role is unlikely to be sufficient in itself nor to be based on traditional respect for professionals alone. This example, moreover, shows that general terms such as 'Asian' can also be problematic in analyses of culture (see comments above about the plurality of Western cultures also).

So far this discussion has avoided the more underlying ethical issue of whether it is possible or desirable to attempt to find universal values and principles or whether cultural diversity requires a relativistic response. These matters are addressed in detail in Chapters 4, 5 and 6. However, at this point it is necessary to acknowledge that the hypothetical examples used here to examine aspects of cultural differences also point to this issue. Are the Botshoma family's views about the discipline of children simply different to the mainstream Western context in which they now live or are they mistaken about children's rights? Does Shu-Mei have a greater understanding than Geoff of the dilemma facing Jill about care for her mother and, if so, should this affect the assessment? (We might also ask if any difference of view between Shu-Mei and Geoff is influenced by gender.) Is it necessary to think of values and ethics in social work and the human services as being basically different between cultures and countries or should we try to find a way to ensure that shared ethical documents and discussions identify the values and ethics that make an international professional discourse possible? These are questions that can be answered both from universal and from culturally relative perspectives, but as has been shown by this discussion the answers that would be given would have quite markedly different implications for how 'good' practice and policy can be conceived.

It is also necessary at this point to note that the hypothetical examples above are both located in Western contexts. One of them concerns service users who have migrated from another country and the other a professional practitioner who also is a migrant, both identifiable in these settings as members of ethnic minorities. In that sense they both relate to 'international social work' as that is increasingly recognized (Healy, 2008; Hugman, 2010). The ethical issues raised here are likely also to be encountered by Western social workers and other human services practitioners going to practice in non-Western settings and by others moving between different contexts (Gray, 2005; Healy, 2008). Questions of cultural difference in values and ethics can also relate to the situations of those who are members of long-standing ethnic minority communities and also of Indigenous peoples, whether as service users or professionals. Socio-economic class may also constitute cultural differences between service users and professionals (this point is developed further in Chapter 5). It might be thought that this affects countries that are 'multicultural' compared to those that are not. Certainly the literature in social work and the human services about this issue tends to be from Western countries, whether in Europe or the settler countries. To the extent that this is the case it may be considered as an aftermath of empire, with ethnic minority communities often comprised of people whose family origins lie in the countries that were colonized. However, the ethnic diversity of populations and the presence of ethnic minorities, including Indigenous peoples, is not confined to the post-colonial Western countries. Social workers and other human services practitioners in many countries will have to work with people who are from a different culture to their own. But it is also the case that social work as a profession and modern approaches to human services more generally developed originally in Western countries (Payne, 2005; Hugman, 2010). As these concepts and practices were adopted in other parts of the world Western theories and perspectives have continued to dominate international debate, although there is some recent development of locally authentic ('indigenized') approaches (Razack, 2000; Gray & Fook, 2004; Gray, 2005; Healy, 2008; Hugman, 2010). So it may be said that through the conscious development of social work and other aspects of Western social welfare in non-Western countries, as well as the involvement of Western social workers and other human services practitioners in international social development work, the challenges of cross-cultural values and ethics in these practices and policies have become increasingly global (Gray, 2005).

This chapter has examined the way in which questions of cultural difference are central to understanding value and ethics in social work and human services practice and policy. Using two hypothetical case situations it has been argued that values can vary between cultural points of reference and that these affect how practice situations can be understood. It has been noted also that there are broad shared values for social work, in particular, that have an impact on the way in which debates about ethics and values occur in this occupational field. This chapter has alluded to the way in which such questions concern the role of values and ethics in understanding the construction of these occupations as professions, with discrete areas of skill, knowledge and sets of socially mandated responsibilities. So it is to examining the relationship of culture to professionalism and professional ethics that the discussion now turns in the next chapter.

3 Professionalism and ethics in social work and human services

The idea of 'profession', its history and (dis)contents

A significant feature of any analysis of social work and the human services is the complex pattern of professionalization in the field. Globally, social work is the most highly professionalized of the social welfare occupations, but even that varies between countries. Moreover, in some countries there has been a long-standing critical position among some social workers against the pursuit of professional status (for example, compare Reisch & Andrews, 2002, with Olson, 2007). Similarly, community workers, youth workers, social care workers and others demonstrate ambivalence about claims to professional status (Mendes, 2002; Butcher *et al.*, 2007; Banks, 2010; Sercombe, 2010).

To understand why there should be ambivalence about professionalization in these fields it is necessary to ask why occupations pursue professionalism; what are the benefits and problems of this way of constructing such occupations? The classic answer to this question is that a profession is a particular type of occupation (Greenwood, 1957; Carr-Saunders & Wilson, 1962; Etzioni, 1969). In this view, professions are distinguished by certain characteristics, or 'traits', that separate them from other occupations. The exact lists of core traits varies according to the criteria used in different analyses, but common features include a high level of specialized skills and a knowledge base that are largely unique to the occupation, self-control over the occupation (including how it is defined, who can be regarded as a member, what counts as appropriate practice and so on), authority for the occupation sanctioned by the wider community and a code of ethics that provides a basis for trust between professionals and their clientele. In many ways this approach has similarities with the wider 'everyday' idea of a profession as an occupation that is somehow different or even 'special' in comparison to other types of work. Seen in this way, the concept can be regarded as a theorization of 'common sense' (Freidson, 1983a). On the basis of this approach, Etzioni and his colleagues (for example, Toren, 1972) propose the notion of 'semi-profession' to describe social work and human services, as well as nursing, allied health, school teaching and so on. These occupations, they argue, cannot by their very nature achieve all of the key characteristics of the 'full' or 'classic' professions, such as medicine, dentistry, law, religious ministry or architecture.

The trait approach has been criticized extensively on several grounds. First, it can be seen as a circular argument, in that the criteria used are derived from empirical studies of those occupations that have been successful historically in establishing claims to professional status, especially medicine and law (Hugman, 1991, p. 3). Thus the internal logic of the argument has the structure of saying 'a profession is an occupation that has the characteristics of occupational forms that are regarded as professions'. More substantively, criticisms of trait theory point to the centrality of occupational self-control and high social status as the social characteristics that set these occupations apart from others (Johnson, 1972; Wilding, 1982). Freidson (1983a, p. 19) notes that some critical analysis has called professions 'privileged private governments'. From this analysis, claims to esoteric skills and knowledge and to distinctive ethics are understood as serving the purpose of being political strategies for 'occupational closure'; that is, they are used to mark out the boundaries of an occupation and to control those who are admitted to membership.

The second ground for criticizing the trait theory of professions is that it obscures the importance of gender in the historical construction of these occupations (Hugman, 1991; Witz, 1992; Weeks, 1995; Davies, 1996). The classic theories simply do not notice that the professions had been exclusive to men for a long time and even by the end of the twentieth century were still overwhelmingly dominated by men. In contrast, the so-called semi-professions historically were women's professions. Even when this is noticed, for example by Toren (1972), the explanation offered is that this is because of the nature of women, as opposed to a more critical analysis of gender segregation as a social process. Similarly, as the critique of professions and patriarchy gained influence, other social segregations started to be recognized, in particular those of ethnicity and 'race', disability and sexuality (Stubbs, 1985; Oliver, 1990; Hugman, 1991; Jackson, 1995; Weeks, 1995). (It can be observed that even in this analysis the question of age discrimination is still largely addressed in terms of older service users, as opposed to older members of professions.) The problem with professionalization, as it is understood from this perspective, is that it appears largely to serve the interest of the professionals and, moreover, of particular social groups within the professions.

So it may be argued that ambivalence towards the idea of professionalization in social work and the human services is founded on the core values that are claimed by these occupations, namely human rights and social justice. These values, especially the latter with strong elements of egalitarianism, challenge those social processes that would demarcate professionals from service users. The problems which human services address are those that might affect any person, in the sense that they are expressions of the human condition (compare with Nussbaum, 2001). What differentiates human service professionals from their clientele is not a social superiority but rather the possession of particular skills and knowledge, combined with social roles (for example, as employees of social service agencies) which provide the basis for helping.

One possible way of addressing the power of professionals has been to create a 'market' relationship in service provision, through which service users are empowered to make choices as consumers (Parton, 1994; Hugman, 1998; Stark, 2010). Where service users are able to exercise this type of power then, it is argued, professionals as the producers of services must be more responsive. Yet there are also significant weaknesses in the market model, of which the most important is that professional services of these kinds are 'produced' at the point of 'consumption' (Hugman, 1998). Consumer goods, such as cars, televisions and so on exist independently of the producer or the consumer, whereas professional services are actions occurring between people. Added to this, the focus or content of such services is people themselves, in the sense of practice being directed to effecting change in individuals, families or communities (their identity or self, their relationships, their functioning and so on) as well as in their social environments. Furthermore, such services are most often 'produced' through an interpersonal relationship of some kind. So the dynamic that may exist in the purchase of consumer goods or other types of service cannot operate in the same way (Hugman, 1998; Stark, 2010; compare with Freidson, 2001, p. 65). This argument lends weight to the claim that the more important factors underlying the attempts to shift to market models in social welfare are political and economic. That is, cost reduction has been a major goal of governments in the last two decades and controlling the practices of professionals in the health and social welfare fields has been a major strategy towards this overall objective (Flaherty *et al.*, 2008). This movement has been buttressed by a particular set of political values, notably a distinctive new form of liberalism, hence 'neo-liberalism', in which each individual is held to have complete moral responsibility for all aspects of their lives and so must be given total responsibility for making the necessary arrangements to achieve their own vision of what is good. Not only is this intended to lead to 'small government', but also to limit the authority of professions. It is 'privatization' both in the sense of selling government entities into private ownership and at the same time emphasizing the private responsibility of each citizen for her or his own well-being (Carey, 2008; Liljegren *et al.*, 2008; Chan & Wang, 2009).

In response to these pressures, professions have sought to demonstrate more tangibly that their practices are effective and efficient (Smith, 2004). This move is usually referred to as 'evidence-based', in that the emphasis is on being able to provide clear evidence as to why particular practices should be used to address specific problems and why any one profession should be seen as the appropriate one to be providing this service. As Macdonald and Macdonald (1995), Thyer (2007) and others argue, there is an ethical basis for such an approach, in that if a practice is not known to be the best or most appropriate then using it is not morally defensible. At the same time, a suspicion has grown that the use of 'evidence-based' criteria has easily become harnessed to the project of professional boundary maintenance rather than ethical accountability to service users. Indeed, it is noteworthy that such concerns about the emphasis on 'evidence-based practice' have often displaced other concerns about professionalization in the social work and human service literature in the first decade of the twenty-first century (Smith, 2004; Dominelli & Holloway, 2008).

However, recent studies of professionalization point to the impact of these criti-cisms and debates in ways that have led not to the abandonment of professionalism but instead to the emergence of a 'new professionalism' (Freidson, 1994; Davies, 1996; Irvine, 2001; Svensson, 2006; Leicht *et al.*, 2009). This approach to profes-sionalism seeks to be more democratic, in the sense of recognizing that service users are actors in the service relationship, they are subjects who engage in a relationship through which assistance is provided (Hugman, 1991, 1998; Øvretveit *et al.*, 1997; Beresford, 2000; Willumsen & Skivenes, 2005; Leung, 2010). Embedded in this understanding there is also a moral claim: the focus of practice is the lives of service users and not the skills and knowledge of professionals (Koehn, 1994). Therefore the skills and knowledge of professionals have value in so far as they are able to assist in resolving social problems or helping people to improve their lives, not in or of themselves.

One way of understanding the changes in the professions brought about by these developments is the concept of 'deprofessionalization' (Derber, 1987). This concept refers to the way in which professionals increasingly have been employed within large organizations, whether government, not-for-profit or for-profit, providing health and social welfare services (Cousins, 1987). Professionals within such organizations, it is argued, become effectively a very highly specialized workforce, with considerable discretion in the use of skill and knowledge, but with the trade-off that the overall objectives of their work are set by organizational policy. If, as earlier analyses of professionalization had argued, occupational control and autonomy were the key goals, then consumer-focused markets and evidence-based practice could be said to point (perhaps negatively) in this direction. However, Freidson (1983b, 1984, 1994), although for a long time a severe critic of the professions (see above), has increasingly argued against this concept is an over-interpretation of social change. He points to the fact that it is often senior professionals who set organizational objectives and manage their junior colleagues; or at least senior professionals have a significant role in such goal setting perhaps in partnership with other managers and policy makers (1984, p. 12; 2001). For Freidson, another important change has been that profes-sions are now clearly segmented so that the ancient 'fiction' of equality of authority and esteem has been rapidly eroded (1984, p. 15). Dent (1999) agrees, asserting that the more accurate way to understand this process is to see it as a way of enhancing the collective autonomy of an occupation at the cost of the individual autonomy of practitioners at the level of direct service provision.

For Freidson (1994), whose careful but critical analysis now seems quite prescient, the goal of such critique and debate should be that professionalism is 'reborn' through focusing on the ethical commitment to service. Freidson's (2001) last major contribution to this debate is constructed around the idea that it is the *ethical* dimen-sion of professionalism that provides the main point at which service users can make claims on professions, because the value of service can only be realized at this point: in other words, in practice. So the main challenge to professionalism is that which seeks to remove or deny the ethical commitment to the goals of service, partnership with service users and other democratic forms of practice (Hugman, 1998; Dent,

1999; Beresford, 2000; Freidson, 2001; Irvine, 2001; Svensson, 2006; compare with Bauman, 1994). Such a view leads to the concept of a 'new professionalism', one that is grounded in the ability of professions to open themselves up to partnership models in their relationships with service users both individually and in the form of representative groups (Beresford, 2000; Healy & Meagher, 2004; Maidment, 2006; Postle & Beresford, 2007; Scourfield, 2007; compare with Hugman, 1991). As Beresford (2000) makes clear, for such a model of professionalism to be a reality it has to go beyond the type of token relationship that is inherent in consumerism. Maidment (2006) uses the term 'alliance' to convey the difference, implying that this is a relationship that is based on mutuality and one which continues over a period of time (also see Postle & Beresford, 2007). For this reason, just as the capacity of service users to gain power in relation to professions is greater when approached collectively (Hugman, 1991), so too are professionals more likely to be able to develop and sustain such relationships when acting together. In so far as the analysis of professionalism as hierarchical is correct, and accepting that most professional work in the human services field occurs in organizations, the capacity for such a model to be realized at the level of everyday practice requires that professional organizations provide the ethical basis for this approach. Thus, it is for this reason that a major aspect of the potential for professions to develop democratic practices lies in their capacity to develop and assert ethical frameworks, independently of employing organizations. In this sense, present day challenges can be seen as very similar to those facing social work and related fields in their earliest days (compare with Addams, 2002 [1907]).

Is professionalization a cultural phenomenon?

So far in this discussion, the issues identified and the arguments that have been summarized have arisen in those parts of the word where social work, youth work, community work and other human services occupations first began to professionalize and social welfare services became institutionalized in modern forms. In other words, these are debates that largely draw on developments in Western countries. Freidson (1983a, p. 22) goes so far as to declare that 'profession' is 'a changing historic concept, with particular roots in ... industrial nation[s] strongly influenced by Anglo-American traditions'. This seems to be reasonably accurate because, as has already been noted in Chapters 1 and 2, social work and human services have developed out of this context to become an increasingly world-wide form of response to social and personal welfare needs. This has partly been as a consequence of globalization, in which ideas and practices are increasingly exchanged around the world, but also because as countries have developed economically they have faced the same challenges as those that were encountered in the global North, namely the social impacts of industrialization and mass urbanization, with associated 'modernization' of social structures and relationships (such as changing patterns of family life). Some analysts suggest that globalization in this sense represents 'Westernization' of social structures and culture (Ritzer, 2000).

However, in the same way that contemporary forms of professionalization in global Northern countries are in many ways profoundly different to the forms that existed there in previous centuries, it might be expected that forms of professionalization in other parts of the world will also have distinctive features. The debates summarized above have taken place within the context of a liberal world-view, after an extended historical period of the rise of rationalism and democratic law as the bases for public life. Recognizing this historical circumstance, the question is raised as to whether the path of professionalization in other parts of the world must necessarily be the same, even though many professions now identify themselves as global. This includes social work, youth work, community work and other human services professions, as much as it does medicine, dentistry, nursing, allied health and the remedial therapies, or even law, accountancy and engineering.

To a great extent there is evidence that broad features of professionalism in social work and human services are common across the various parts of the world (for example, compare: Mafile'o, 2004 [Tonga/Aotearoa-New Zealand]; Templeman, 2004 [Russia]; Carten & Goodman, 2005 [Caribbean]; Osei-Hwedie *et al.*, 2006 [Botswana]; Yan & Cheung, 2006 [China]; Hugman *et al.*, 2007 [Vietnam]; Lin & Wang, 2010 [Taiwan]). The traits of professions described by earlier studies are still apparent, in the form of recognized education and training, professional organizations with criteria for membership and codes of ethics, and in some countries legislative sanction for particular groups to practice. What appears to be the most common element among these is systematic education and training, at college and university level, which in many analyses is addressed as if this alone constitutes professionalization. This is not to suggest that education and training are not important, as there is widespread agreement that skilled practices do require development as well as being supported and tested by systematic knowledge. The point is that this element of professionalization appears to be the common feature between most countries as well as between the various human services occupations and at times can be seen as the principal or even sole marker of professionalization. (The discussion returns to this point below.)

These processes have often been encouraged and supported by international organizations including both international professional bodies and also non-government organizations, such as UNICEF, UNDP and a variety of other more issue specific independent agencies (Cox & Pawar, 2006; Healy, 2008; Hugman, 2010). Indeed, in some countries such models have been deliberately 'imported' from other (usually Western) locations because they are regarded as having been comparatively successful in achieving the goal of professionalization. It seems reasonable to suggest that such a trend is part of the wider processes of globalization. Moreover, as the transfer of ideas is almost exclusively from Western countries to other parts of the world elements of neo-colonialism must be considered. The international organizations that promote and support professionalization in this sector are not neutral, in the sense that they control access to resources and therefore can exert strong influence on those countries that require developmental assistance. This is as much the case in the social welfare sector as it is in relation to the economy or infrastructural development. The distinction of global North and South, first proposed by the Brandt Commission (1980), continues to have some relevance here as it implicitly distinguishes between the countries where social work and human services first professionalized and those in which this process is part of wider on-going social development.

Two examples from the global South demonstrate the variations in ways of understanding professionalization and professionalism: Botswana and China. To begin with the instance of Botswana, Osei-Hwedie (1993) argues that the process of professionalization in human services has been dominated by a post-colonial view of social work. Consequently it has been necessary to rethink both the boundaries of that particular profession as well as the cultural relevance of some aspects of the structures and content inherited from the British colonial era. This represents a process that has also been described elsewhere (see comments on China below) and was first discussed in relation to the modernization of social work in Egypt from a colonial model to a more culturally appropriate form. This is the approach of 'indigenization' (making the profession relevant to the indigenous context: adapting external ideas to fit local circumstances) and 'authentization' (locating and building on authentic foundations in local social structures and relationships: creating a genuinely 'domestic model' of practice and policy) (Walton & El Nasr, 1988, pp. 148–149). The actual structure of professional education that has resulted in Botswana has many similarities with global Northern models, but the content is grounded in local culture and social institutions (Osei-Hwedie *et al.*, 2006). In particular, the predominant emphasis is on social and community development as the central goal of practice. Although the definition of social work used in Botswana can be seen as having clear similarities with that used in the USA (Osei-Hwedie *et al.*, 2006, p. 573), it concentrates on effecting change in social circumstances and developing appropriate action for social and community development rather than on individual capacities and social functioning (compare with Patel, 2005). In particular, the curriculum is related to government policy as representing the overall needs and priorities of the society. In addition, the government is a major employer in human services and so provides authority for these occupations. The outcome is a culturally and structurally relevant form of education. In addition, there is a series of levels of education, with a Diploma, Bachelors degree and Masters degree integrating in sequence. The Diploma and Bachelors levels are generalist, with a strong social and community development focus and including youth work, disability services, probation, community health and other related service areas. The MSW level emphasizes policy, research, management, education and training and professional development. In this way, the shape of professionalization has many similarities with the global North but at the same time not only is built on local knowledge and practice methods but also takes a broader and less differentiated approach to the boundaries of social work, community development, youth work and other human service practices.

The process of professionalization in China began more recently but has progressed very rapidly. In this setting there has also been a deliberate strategy of using indigenization and authentization to create social work and human services that are internationally recognizable but at the same time have Chinese characteristics (Yeun-Tsang & Sung, 2002; Yan & Cheung, 2006; Tsang *et al.*, 2008). Here too higher level education and training is the central element in professionalization. However, there are two major differences from the situation in Botswana. First, the way in which professions are constructed within the Chinese political system gives the government a greater direct controlling role in the organization and the content of social work and human services. Not only does an occupation require government approval, in the form of law and policy decision, to exist at all but also the government must sanction the leadership of a profession, its educational curriculum and so on. Second, there is a clear distinction between the economically developed east of China and the developing west in the forms of social work and human services that are being created. In the east human services are predominantly provided by the Ministry of Civil Affairs, taking forms that would be recognizable in many global Northern countries. That is, these are social welfare services that focus on the needs of individuals, families and groups within the community. They encompass family and child-care problems, social needs arising from physical and mental health issues, disabilities, community corrections and problems associated with old age. In contrast, in western China there is a much greater need for community development approaches that reflect the social and economic issues that face whole communities (Yuen-Tsang & Sung, 2002; Tsang *et al.*, 2008). Nevertheless, across China a very similar overall process of professionalization is evident as in other parts of the world.

When these developments are compared, it would appear that there are very close similarities between the route taken to professionalization in Botswana and China and that of the global North. Although there are clearly issues of globalization and neo-colonialism, these two examples also point to the way in which these forces are not so determining that they prevent the pursuit of indigenized and authentic forms of professions that are relevant to different contexts. Of particular note here is the emphasis on finding appropriate ways of linking the goals and the methods of practice, so that relevant 'ends' are pursued by relevant 'means'. While these factors are made tangible in the form of institutions, policies and so on, they also indicate the centrality of grounding the 'ethos' of the professions concerned in that of the culture, or cultures, of each country. This means that attention must be given not only to how social work, youth work, community work and other human services are undertaken, but how they are organized, through which agencies their services are provided, and even how or if distinctions are drawn between them. As has already been noted in the preceding chapters, in some contexts the term 'social work' is used synonymously for all human services, while in others distinctions are made between this and youth work, community work and so on.

To the extent that Freidson (1994, 2001) is correct that ethics is central to the idea and the reality of professionalism, it is important also to ask about this element alongside factors such as specialized education and employment structures. In this respect we can find a wide variation in approaches taken. For Osei-Hwedie and his colleagues (2006), as well as for others writing about African social work, ethics tends to be considered as a question of cultural values before it is anything else (also see Silavwe, 1995; compare with Dove, 2010). What is necessary, it is argued, is for the nature of social work and human services to be considered from the perspective of an African world-view, with a strong emphasis on communality and mutuality (Graham, 2002). Similar approaches can be seen in other parts of the world, for example in the Pacific Island cultures (Mafile'o, 2004, 2006).

In Asia the role of ethics in the processes of professionalization appears to be somewhat different, at least on the face of it. As a topic it appears to be relatively little discussed, with reasons for this divided into three themes. First, many Asian countries have long traditions of public officials, whose actions were guided by ethical principles, but these were usually part of cultural expectations and not separately codified. To some extent there are parallels with the notion of virtue in Western ethics, although Lai (2006) questions this comparison. As modernized forms of professions have gained prominence, along with industrialization and other related changes, the approach of developing codes of ethics has been widely adopted as part of the necessary structures and systems (Lin & Wang, 2010). Second, when Asian human services professionals identify ethics as an important question it is more likely to be in relation to the value conflict experienced by service users between tradition and contemporary social life (Doe *et al.*, 2009; Feng *et al.*, 2009). In some circumstances, professionals may also themselves feel a struggle between tradition and the expectations of a modern code of ethics. This tends to emphasize the understanding of ethics as a set of rules for professional conduct. Third, in some circumstances a formal systematization of ethics may be considered as inappropriate. Weiss-Gal and Welbourne (2008, p. 287) note that in India there is not a nationally accepted national code of ethics for social work, for example. From a slightly different point of view, Yip (2004) has challenged the use of Western ethical principles in Chinese social work as a failure of indigenization, which can actually lead to bad practice because of cultural inappropriateness.

Taking an international comparative view of the role of ethics in professionalization raises questions about whether it has come to be regarded as a technical matter, reflecting the mechanistic dynamic in a trait approach to professions that having identified the necessary elements then seeks to assemble them. Yet, as the concern with the relationship between knowledge, skills and values evident in all of these contexts demonstrates, ethics is not only a technical question but also one that goes to the heart of the nature of social work and human services. In Chapter 1 ethics was defined as the conscious reflection on moral values, but in many cases the use of ethics has run the risk of rendering it a technique or device necessary for an occupation to professionalize. As noted in the earlier chapter, this can then conflate ethics with 'codes of conduct' as opposed to it being the on-going discourse on the ethos of a profession. For this reason, it is not a problem that Banks (2006) identifies some key differences in the social work codes of ethics of 31 countries that she reviewed; rather it should be regarded positively as the product of cultural differences and the appropriate variations in moral concerns that are held in different parts of the world.

The challenge for social work and the human services is to be able to think about ethics internationally and cross-culturally. It is certainly the case that much of the considered discussion of professional ethics in this field is 'Western', in the sense of coming from Western Europe and North America (as defined by Osei-Hwedie *et al.*, 2006, p. 581). Although it is necessary to note that even this way of examining the world can tend to obscure cultural differences (as does speaking of 'Africa' and 'Asia'), in the broadest terms this is an accurate observation. So, how can social work and human services address professional ethics internationally and cross-culturally in ways that recognize cultural diversity while also holding to a shared notion of this field and the professions within it? This is the question to which this chapter now turns.

The international ethics debate

To look in more detail at the international aspects of professional ethics, this discussion focuses on social work. As the most widely professionalized human services occupation internationally, it provides a clear example of the issues that have been identified. In fact, in the form of the International Federation of Social Workers (IFSW) and the International Association of Schools of Social Work (IASSW), social work can be described as an internationally organized profession. These two organizations share an ethical document, *Ethics in Social Work: Statement of Principles* (IFSW/IASSW, 2004). Their partner organization, the International Council on Social Welfare (ICSW), which represents the interests of human services, social development and social policy more widely, does not share authorship of this statement (although it refers to it when it wants to address the topic). There is no comparable international organization covering youth work, community work, social development work, social care work or others in human services, although ICSW does relate to some aspects of these fields. The health professions, such as medicine, nursing and psychology, do have comparable international bodies that each have their own ethical statements, such as the international code of ethics for nursing (ICN, 2006) and the 'universal declaration' of ethics for psychology (IUPS, 2008).

The ethical statement of the IFSW and IASSW consists of several parts. First, it introduces the purpose of an ethical statement and makes links with the definition of social work (see Chapter 1). The introduction makes it clear that the statement is intended to be quite general and to present core values in order to 'encourage social workers across the world to reflect on the challenges and dilemmas that face them and to make ethical decisions' (sec. 1). It also makes links to background international documents such as the *Universal Declaration of Human Rights* (UN, 1948) and other declarations and conventions (sec. 3). The following section (sec. 4) sets out the two foundational principles, human rights and social justice. Each of these is briefly defined and then subsidiary points are made about more detailed aspects of them. It is this section that may be considered as the core of the document; some applied points are then spelled out in section 5, where it is considered that sufficient international agreement exists (for example, prohibiting social workers being involved in torture or terrorism, sec. 5.2).

4.1   Human Rights and Human Dignity

Social work is based on respect for the inherent worth and dignity of all people, and the rights that follow from this. Social workers should uphold and defend each person's physical, psychological, emotional and spiritual integrity and well-being. This means:

1. Respecting the right to self-determination – Social workers should respect and promote people's right to make their own choices and decisions, irrespective of their values and life choices, provided this does not threaten the rights and legitimate interests of others.
2. Promoting the right to participation – Social workers should promote the full involvement and participation of people using their services in ways that enable them to be empowered in all aspects of decisions and actions affecting their lives.
3. Treating each person as a whole – Social workers should be concerned with the whole person, within the family, community, societal and natural environments, and should seek to recognise all aspects of a person's life.
4. Identifying and developing strengths – Social workers should focus on the strengths of all individuals, groups and communities and thus promote their empowerment.

4.2.   Social Justice

Social workers have a responsibility to promote social justice, in relation to society generally, and in relation to the people with whom they work. This means:

1. Challenging negative discrimination* – Social workers have a responsibility to challenge negative discrimination on the basis of characteristics such as ability, age, culture, gender or sex, marital status, socio-economic status, political opinions, skin colour, racial or other physical characteristics, sexual orientation, or spiritual beliefs. *In some countries the term "discrimination" would be used instead of "negative discrimination". The word negative is used here because in some countries the term "positive discrimination" is also used. Positive discrimination is also known as "affirmative action". Positive discrimination or affirmative action means positive steps taken to redress the effects of historical discrimination against the groups named in clause 4.2.1 above.
2. Recognising diversity – Social workers should recognise and respect the ethnic and cultural diversity of the societies in which they practise, taking account of individual, family, group and community differences.
3. Distributing resources equitably – Social workers should ensure that resources at their disposal are distributed fairly, according to need.
4. Challenging unjust policies and practices – Social workers have a duty to bring to the attention of their employers, policy makers, politicians and the general public situations where resources are inadequate or where distribution of resources, policies and practices are oppressive, unfair or harmful.
5. Working in solidarity – Social workers have an obligation to challenge social conditions that contribute to social exclusion, stigmatisation or subjugation, and to work towards an inclusive society.

Box 3.1 **Excerpt from** *Ethics in Social Work: Statement of Principles*, **section 4 (IFSW/IASSW, 2004)**

Although these principles and the detailed application of them are derived from international documents, the approach of having a single shared statement for social work globally is not universally accepted. Just as the *Universal Declaration of Human Rights* is perceived by some critics as an imposition of global Northern values on other countries and cultures (summarized, for example, by Gasper, 2006), so too in social work the idea of an international statement has been questioned on the same grounds (Weaver, 1997; Gray & Fook, 2004; Yip, 2004; Gray, 2005; Mafile'o, 2006; Green & Baldry, 2008). There is considerable diversity also among these critics, as some would prefer to see no such statement, some challenge particular aspects (such as the idea of 'universal' human rights or the specification of particular rights), while others would prefer a greater sense of 'cultural humility' and more of an attempt to be integrative of values and principles that come from global Southern positions.

Yet none of the critics of the statement, or aspects of it, appears to be suggesting that it is totally impossible to discuss social work as an internationally recognizable set of ideas and practices. There are those who are concerned about whether this is part of a neo-colonial misconception about how social work might be defined, in other words that the ethical statement reflects a global Northern view of the nature of social work (Gray & Fook, 2004; Yip, 2004; Gray, 2005; Mafile'o, 2006; Green & Baldry, 2008). However, this should not be taken as an argument for understanding social work as inherently so different in each context that it cannot be discussed internationally or cross-culturally (compare with Weiss, 2005). What is being sought from this critical perspective is a more inclusive view of social work, one that will permit difference and diversity to be grasped and accommodated.

A statement of ethical principles such as the IFSW/IASSW document can be understood at two levels. One is that of substantive, or applied ethics, which concerns the detail of each article. Debate at this level focuses on whether matters such as participation, a holistic approach, challenging discrimination or equity are indeed the core expressions of the principles of human rights and human dignity and social justice in social work and human services. The second level is that of normative ethics, which asks whether the principles of human rights and human dignity and social justice are the foundations of ethics in this field as a whole. In the following chapters both these levels are seen to play a crucial role in the analysis of culture in relation to professional values and ethics. Banks (2006, p. 41) argues that this is to be expected, referring to such an apparent mixing of principles that have different philosophical foundations as 'common morality'. This implies both that such an approach is part of everyday morality, shared widely within society, and also that it is grounded in what is common between principles rather than their differences. The philosophical position that underpins such an approach is that of 'ethical pluralism', to which this discussion returns in Chapter 6.

Given the close relationship between social work and other human services fields, with relatively permeable boundaries as has been noted above, it is not surprising that fields such as youth work, social development and community work, social care and so on share the same range of value positions. Indeed, in youth work (Banks & Imam, 2000; Sercombe, 2010), social development and community work (Reisch & Lowe, 2000; Mendes, 2002; Hardina, 2004; Munford & Walsh-Tapiata, 2006) and social care (Lloyd, 2010) the same broad principles are considered and debated. Not only have these professional groups emerged in the same period and the same societies but also they share similar objectives and methods (ends and means). (The same point can be noted with regard to the international ethical documents of medicine, nursing, psychology [WMA, 2005; ICN, 2006; IUPS, 2008].) So for this reason the issues raised by the international ethics framework of social work can form the beginning point for the analysis of ethics in the human services more generally. How these issues then appear in more detail will be seen to differ between the context and orientation of practitioners and of services as well as between countries and cultures.

Conclusion

Debates about cultural difference in values return the discussion to the question noted in Chapter 1 concerning how we can make judgements between positions that can simply be seen as 'different' and circumstances when it might be reasonable to argue that a position is 'wrong' (compare with Hinman, 2008). To this might be added whether it is possible to have a profession with an ethics that can embrace diversity while at the same time providing a shared set of core values. The discussion in this chapter has identified ethics as a central feature of professionalization, not simply as a mechanism that enables an occupation to claim the status of 'profession' but because it also enables occupations to articulate the relationship between the ends and means of their practices. In this way, it has been argued, occupations that work with aspects of people's selves, their families and their communities, and whose work must be constantly negotiated as it is undertaken, are able to be accountable and responsible to those who use their services.

   International and cross-cultural challenges to a shared ethics point social work and human services professionals to an important debate in ethics, namely that between universalist and relativist positions. The former argue that because people share a common humanity, core moral values and issues are basically the same; in other words, they are universal. The latter take the opposite view, asserting that all values are relative to the person or group who hold those values. (As will be seen, this position subdivides into ethical relativism and cultural relativism, which have some important differences.) How the relationship between culture, values and ethics in social work and human services is understood will be crucially affected by whether a universalist or relativist position is taken, So in the next two chapters the discussion focuses in turn on each of these, before then going on to look at a third position, pluralism, that seeks to move beyond the binary implications of this debate.

4   Universal values and ethics

What are universal values?

In the preceding chapters reference has been made to the way in which values and ethics are shared across various professional and occupational groupings within the human services field, along with related areas such as health and education. It has also been noted that internationally the same sorts of statement are made about these matters. This degree of commonality suggests a high level of agreement in modern societies about those things that are important and how they should be achieved. The documents that set out the value positions and the ethics of these various professional groupings are also intended in principle to apply to everyone who is involved in them, without exceptions (Banks, 2006; Bowles *et al.*, 2006). For service users and for others outside these professions, therefore, there ought to be an expectation that such statements are observed by every practitioner with whom they have contact, applied equally to all those to whom they provide a service. So, the predominant view is that professional ethics are 'universal' both in the sense of embodying values that ought to be applied to all work with every service user but also in the way that they place this obligation on all members of the profession or occupation in question.

In this chapter the approach of 'universalism' is examined. First, universalism is explained briefly and its connections with contemporary social work and human services are discussed. In particular, the ways in which the values of human rights and social justice are understood are shown to have strong universal features. Some problems in applying universalism in practice are then identified. This leads to a deeper discussion of the way in which the idea of universalism has developed, which in turn is followed by the introduction of some examples of important ways in which recent arguments about social well-being have sought to maintain the value of humanity as something shared by all people.

A claim to the universal nature of professional values and ethics can be seen in the following situation.

Maria is a woman in her mid-twenties who was born in the Sudan but is now living as a refugee settled permanently in a Western country. She has two children who are both attending primary school. Maria is in the process of getting divorced from her husband, who is also from the Sudan. They arrived in their new country after separate journeys from their home region and they both blame the break-up of their relationship on the traumas that they experienced while fleeing from the civil war. The principal at her children's school has suggested to Maria that she should ask for assistance from the local child welfare agency because she is finding it hard to cope with looking after the children. Maria is reluctant to do this because she has experienced some negative attitudes from staff in some of the welfare agencies that she has had contact with in the settlement process, which she felt were because of her different racial and cultural background and that she is a refugee. Maria is surprised when the principal explains that the professionals at the child welfare agency, like teachers, have a code of ethics that states they should treat all people with respect and seek to provide them with appropriate help whatever their cultural background. But she feels reassured when the principal says 'they start from the fact that we are all human beings and we all have the same rights – so you should expect them to help you in the same way that they would help anyone else. It's just like the way that we care the same for all the children in the school.'

The approach that is being described here is one that is grounded in the idea of universal values and ethics. As this senior teacher states, it is based on the idea that all human beings have the same moral value. In other words, in terms of ethics, people should all be considered equal. So for a young mother such as Maria, whether she receives assistance should not depend on her national or cultural origin, her 'racial' identity, her sex or her age, or any other factor except the needs that she has.

Underpinning this approach is the view that all human beings have the same basic characteristics in common: the core of what it is 'to be human' is shared by everyone. A key idea grounded in this view that has been particularly influential in social work and human services is the theory of human needs proposed by Maslow (1970). The basis of Maslow's approach is a social psychology of human personality and motivation, in which he considered how people's lives are shaped by the needs that they experience. Maslow's model is a successive hierarchy, in which there is a clear order in which needs must be met. At the most basic is the need for physical survival (water, food, shelter); this is followed in turn by needs for safety and security, for membership of a social group, for love, affection and close relationships and, finally, for the accomplishment of the higher faculties (of thought, creativity, choice and so on, which Maslow calls 'self-actualization'). For Maslow these needs are common to all people and can be considered as central to understanding what it is to be 'fully human' (but compare with Nussbaum, 2001, Part 1, for comment on the implications of more recent research for the extent to which these needs may also be shared to a degree with other animals, especially primates). This model has proved remarkably durable and continues to exert some influence in the theories taught to social work and human services students (Cox & Pawar, 2006).

In Maria's situation it could be said that her needs are currently met at the first and second levels (she has water, food, shelter and she and her children are in a safe place compared to her country of origin). However, Maria's needs at the higher levels are clearly not met and even the psychological aspects of her safety are at risk because of the impact of trauma on her and her husband, as well as the uncertainty of settling somewhere new after fleeing from the country of her birth, the implications of the experience of racism from some people in this new country, and so on. Consequently it can be argued that Maria is not able to 'live well' in her new situation, even though it could be seen as significantly better in many ways than her previous circumstances. Her needs, her capacity to meet them and the values that she and others would use to understand her life are closely interwoven. More importantly, from this perspective all aspects of Maria's situation must be understood in terms of 'what it is to be human' and in this she should not be regarded any differently from anyone else in her new country of residence. From this, she has rights that are the same as everyone else's and so she ought to be enabled to achieve these rights (Ife, 2008).

Universal values in social work and human services ethics

Until quite recently discussions of ethics in social work and human services have tended overwhelmingly to be based on a universal view of human beings and of the values that are held concerning what it is to 'live well'. This can be seen clearly in the claim of international professional organizations that human rights and social justice are foundational principles (IFSW/IASSW, 2004). As noted in the previous chapter, these principles are based on other international documents, especially those that originate from the United Nations. As this body represents 192 countries (at the time of writing), it might be said that the ideas that come from it are 'universal'. This is a contested argument, because against this it can also be argued that certain parts of the world dominate through economic, political and military strength. The position on values that follows from this criticism forms the basis for the discussion in the next chapter. Before that, this chapter looks at the ideas and practices that comprise the universalist position.

The universal view is summed up by the school principal in the illustrative situation described above, that these are values that apply equally to all people. So, if a moral claim is made about one person it must, by definition, apply to everyone. The most obvious example of this is that the human rights set out by the *Universal Declaration of Human Rights* (UN, 1948) are the rights of all human beings in all circumstances. Indeed, Article 1 states 'All human beings are born free and equal in dignity and rights', and Article 2 follows from this, stating:

> Everyone is entitled to all the rights and freedoms set forth in this Declaration, without distinction of any kind, such as race, colour, sex, language, religion, political or other opinion, national or social origin, property, birth or other status. Furthermore, no distinction shall be made on the basis of the political, jurisdictional or international status of the country or territory to which a person belongs, whether it be independent, trust, non-self-governing or under any other limitation of sovereignty.

Articles 3 to 27 then set out in more detail what these rights are, covering such areas as education, health, family and community relationships, and so on. The idea that each person 'ought' to be enabled to achieve these rights is asserted in Article 28: 'Everyone is entitled to a social and international order in which the rights and freedoms set forth in this Declaration can be fully realized.' Article 29 establishes that there are corresponding duties and that the exercise of rights by some people cannot be at the expense of the rights of others. In conclusion, Article 30 states: '[n]othing in this Declaration may be interpreted as implying for any State, group or person any right to engage in any activity or to perform any act aimed at the destruction of any of the rights and freedoms set forth herein.' In a major analysis of human rights in this field, Ife (2008, p. 4) notes that it has direct implications for practice and policy at all levels.

It is this universal view of what it is to be human that forms one of the foundations of ethics in social work and human services (Webster, 2002; Hugman, 2005; Banks, 2006; Bowles *et al.*, 2006; Clifford & Burke, 2009; Sercombe, 2010). Against this view, Webb (2009) argues that the principle of human rights as it has been applied in social work and human services is largely a product of ethical relativism, in that he reads arguments by Briskman (2007), Ife (2008) and others in terms of the way in which they can be seen to place the right to difference and diversity at the centre of their concern. This, Webb states, is not only self-defeating but also undermines the moral claims that social work and human services might make to a concern with cultural differences as a right, which he argues can only be based on seeing 'what it is to be human' as the same for everyone. It leads, he asserts, to social work and human services losing their concern with inequality and disadvantage. (This point is addressed in more detail in Chapter 9.)

The principle of social justice, the other main ethical foundation in this field, is also universal. Bowles *et al.* (2006, p. 110) note that the term has appeared relatively recently in debates and code of ethics, but that the principle itself has informed the field since the late 1800s (also see: Morris, 2002; Reisch, 2002, 2004). This principle is less easily summarized than human rights, because it is 'context dependent' (Bowles *et al.*, 2006, p. 111). However, Bowles and colleagues point to the IFSW/IASSW (2004) statement to argue that it must be taken to signify attention to the way in which inequalities in the distribution of social and material goods affect the lives of all people (some of whom are relatively advantaged while others are disadvantaged). In these terms, social goods include freedom from discrimination and oppression, which may include the distribution of economic opportunities as well as the opportunity to achieve education, health and so on. The importance of addressing discrimination and oppression in relation to these things is that access to them is socially structured through factors such as sex and gender, 'race' and ethnicity, mental and physical (dis)abilities, health, age and so on. These factors affect all people, but in different ways. That is, those who are advantaged must also be considered as they too are affected by such issues.

Much of the present way of thinking about social justice is derived from the work of the political philosopher Rawls (1972). Rawls argues that although there are natural differences in the capacities of individual people, these cannot be considered in any way as 'deserved': the person with natural advantages does not have them because of moral worth, and the same is true for the person who is disadvantaged. So, a society that could be considered just would be one in which the disadvantages arising from such differences would be redressed through policies and practices that would ensure that no-one is treated unequally because of factors over which they have no choice (Reisch, 2002, p. 346). In turn, this points to the way in which a just society must be one that is multicultural (p. 347). Therefore, as Reisch notes, this principle is congruent with universal values in social work and human services that oppose discrimination and oppression and promote equity and diversity. Indeed, on the question of racism and other discriminations of this kind, it should also be noted that any sense of disadvantage arising from difference is a social construct and cannot be seen as natural in the sense meant by Rawls (compare with Dominelli, 2008; Clifford & Burke, 2009).

So, in summary, the universalist position is that the principles of human rights and social justice apply to all people everywhere, not only to some people and/or in some contexts. In Chapter 2 these two principles were seen to be closely intertwined in professional thinking. In fact, in some discussions the two ideas are referred to as a single perspective, even as 'social justice/human rights' (Lundy, 2004, 2006). For Lundy, the concept of need is insufficient to ensure that people will not simply be held responsible for their own problems, when in the situations encountered by social workers and other human services professionals the origins of needs cannot be separated from the unequal distribution of social and material goods. It is only by showing that these are rights that the responsibility of a society can be made explicit.

Statements and codes of ethics take these principles and apply them more concretely to the requirements of what a good practitioner should do in working directly with service users. For many years, at least in English-speaking countries, Biestek's (1957) 'principles of casework' were often taught as professional ethics (for example, see Butrym, 1976). These principles are: individualization; the purposeful expression of feelings; controlled emotional involvement; acceptance (of people as they are); a (morally) non-judgemental attitude; service user self-determination; and confidentiality (p. 89). It is clear that Biestek did not intend them to be generalized as ethics, rather they are proposed in a more technical sense as practice principles specific to voluntary individual counselling and casework (Banks, 2006, p. 35). Nevertheless, some of these can also be taken as ethical principles and appear in both international and national statements and codes, especially non-judgementalism, self-determination and confidentiality (for example: NASW, 1999; YACWA, 2003; IFSW/IASSW, 2004; ICN, 2006; IUPS, 2008; AASW, 2010).

The reason why the sort of practice principles outlined by Biestek should overlap with professional ethics is that they are grounded in the same philosophical approach as that which underpins human rights. This is a perspective that is often summarized as 'respect for persons' (Butrym, 1976; Banks, 2006). The basis for this idea is discussed in greater detail in the next section of this chapter. In professional ethics it tends to be taken as having a practical implication in that each service user, whether they are using services as an individual or as part of a community, should be respected as a unique person who is equally morally valuable as all other persons. From this, it may be said that Maria, in the situation described above, should be treated with such respect by all the service providers with whom she comes into contact, thus making racist or other discriminatory responses quite simply wrong ethically. Furthermore, by working to ensure that practice is not discriminatory service providers are acting on the principle of social justice. Clearly, in an individual case these principles work together to establish a framework for good practice.

Where professional ethics can find that the two principles of human rights and social justice appear potentially to conflict is in the way that human rights unambiguously apply equally to everyone, whereas social justice may require some judgements to be made between who should receive services or assistance. For example, how do human services with limited resources prioritize their responses and select who should receive services, which by implication is a decision that other people will not receive assistance? At the level of practice with individuals or groups the solution to this challenge usually is to develop policies that state what factors are to be taken into account in making such judgements. This takes away the sense that individual practitioners are acting on their own biases, as it allows the terms of a policy to be made public and criteria to be checked against relevant factors about a person, family or group. However, doing this can still be experienced as a conflict between principles, as those who do not receive service may still be seen as 'in need' in terms of other professional theories and concepts. In the case of Maria, that she and her children are treated 'the same' as the other families and children by the school is an expression of respect for persons that embodies their human rights. The family support service that is recommended to Maria by the principal, however, may have to operate on a different basis.

> When Maria arrives at the family support agency for her first visit, she is surprised that early in the conversation the support worker she is talking with, Wendy, tells her that she will have to be assessed to see if she fits the criteria for the service. Maria is not very happy about having to explain her situation in detail before she has got to know the support worker, but Wendy explains that she has to ask Maria some these questions to see if help can be given. After hearing this Maria is confused and asks how this is 'caring for everyone' like the school principal had said. Wendy explains that they do not make judgements about whether to help people based on things like ethnicity, age, disability or sexuality, nor do they make judgements about people being deserving or undeserving of help in a moral sense, but the service does not have enough staff to help everyone so they must work out who is most in need. Although this is not what Maria expected, she decides that if she is going to get help she has to trust Wendy and so she agrees to answer the questions. The agency subsequently decides to provide Maria with assistance, because her status as a single mother, the age of the children and the fact that they are refugees are all seen as priority factors.

This sort of situation is faced by human services and their service users everywhere, even in those countries that have the greatest wealth. In this case Maria receives a service, as do many people, but others approaching this and many agencies also are refused services. If this is because the nature of their problems is not part of the service's remit then it might not be a question of social justice; but often services are having to prioritize because of the level of resources. This can be very challenging for the agency workers who are expected to make decisions about rationing services.

Both the school and the family support agency in this scenario are working with the same broad set of professional ethics. The differences between them arise from other factors. Their purposes, the groups in society that they exist to serve, the way in which they are managed and funded, indeed how much funding they have to do their work, are all factors that affect the way in which questions of human rights and social justice appear to play out in practice. Both are working with a universal view of human rights, in that they apply the same criteria to everyone who seeks to use their services. Both are working with a universal view of social justice, in that they seek not to discriminate against people, for example on grounds of gender or ethnicity. However, the school is expected to serve all the families who live in its area. In contrast, the family support agency is mandated to assist some families, those who require its particular services. Furthermore, it has limited funds and must have ways of deciding who receives help. Therefore, it has to apply social justice principles differently at the level of individual families by actually using these to allocate services.

It is also sometimes argued that good practice requires those in social work and human services to challenge policies that limit the available resources (Dominelli, 2002; Lonne *et al.*, 2004; Olson, 2007). Whether there are sufficient services to help those in need is a social justice issue at the policy level. In global Northern countries, increasingly in the last two decades, the prevailing neo-liberal approach has sought to separate attention to such matters from the way in which services are provided at the level of individuals and families. In ethical terms, however, this weakens or even removes the connection between ends (goals) and means (methods), by emphasizing professional responsibility for the latter while denying professionals a role in making judgements about the former (Mishra, 1987; Hugman, 1998). The ethical challenge that this creates for social work and human services in relation to social justice leads critical commentators to argue that professionals have a moral and political responsibility to oppose and to try to change such policies (Craig, 2002; Ferguson, 2008). This argument refers to that part of the definition of social work in particular that emphasizes pursuing change in social environments, which is also seen in the ethical statements of fields such as youth work and community work (Butcher *et al.*, 2007; Banks, 2010; Sercombe, 2010). From this perspective, while attention to matters such as non-judgmentalism and self-determination are important, they are only one part of the ethics framework. Attention to structural inequality, with resulting discrimination and oppression, is also a central aspect of universal values.

What is the basis for a universal view of values and ethics?

The basis of the ideas that underpin a universal view of values is that of liberalism. As a broad social and political philosophy this is the view that became dominant in global Northern societies by the end of the nineteenth century. Its foundations can be traced several centuries earlier, as European societies were changed by massive upheavals in society, affecting all aspects of life but particularly religion, politics, economics and science. One of the central ideas in this broad movement is that of the freedom of individuals, which was not part of traditional European thought but was fought for over a long period of time.

Of particular note here is the relationship between science and morality. As the influence of religion was challenged by the growth of a variation in belief, philosophers sought to rethink traditional values in a more scientific manner. While many such people contributed to this process, one of the most influential in relation to professional ethics is Kant (Webb & McBeath, 1989; Hugman, 2005; Banks, 2006; Bowles *et al.*, 2006; Beauchamp & Childress, 2009). Kant sought to base ethics on general principles that are independent of an individual's social situation, life commitments and so on, but can be applied in a dispassionate manner in all circumstances. Kant's ethics is based on his understanding of what it is to be human. For him, humanity concerns the moral agency of each person, which derives from a common rationality that separates human beings from the rest of the natural world. Moreover, Kant took a view of humanity that he described as 'cosmopolitanism', in which he argued that the basis of what it is to be human is shared commonly by people in every society (MacIntyre, 1983). To provide a neutral basis for morality, Kant therefore proposes a framework in which 'divine laws' or other culturally grounded notions are replaced by principles of right conduct that apply to everyone and which uphold the human (moral) agency of each person. At the centre of Kant's ethics is the 'categorical imperative' (a principle that is unconditional or absolute), which determines whether a claim about right action made by anyone could be evaluated as achieving this end. The most widely cited version of this imperative statement is that which Kant published in 1785: 'I ought never to act except in such a way that I can also will that my maxim should become a universal law' (Kant, 1964 [1785], p. 67). In other words, any moral claim that I make about an act that I commit must be able to be generalized to every other person. For example, if it is acceptable for me to tell a lie, then I must logically be saying also that it is acceptable for everyone else to do so as well. (This is one of the examples Kant himself uses.) In Kant's approach it is possible to see the echoes of older, religious traditions, especially the statements of the Abrahamic faiths (Judaism, Christianity, Islam) that a good or right action is one that the actor would accept others also committing; the difference is that Kant has removed any reference to divine authority. Morality, for Kant, is grounded in duty to the highest moral principles, hence the term 'deontology' (see discussion in Chapter 1).

The alternative major strand in modern professional ethics is that of utilitarianism. Again as noted in Chapter 1, this is a particular version of the ethics of consequences. For its original proponent, Bentham (1970 [1781]), it is also a way of taking a scientific and rational approach to matters of moral choice. However, where Kant emphasizes duty to a rational principle Bentham proposes a calculation based on the outcomes of acts. Again taking the widely known version of this idea, it argues for the 'greatest happiness of the greatest number (of people)' as the measure of what is good and right (in Freeman, 2000, p. 51). In the original formulation Bentham specifies 'pleasure' as the good which each person would rationally pursue and should be as free as possible to do so, but in response to many criticisms that this is a crude measure, Mill (1910 [1861]) later substitutes the concept of 'happiness'. This latter notion includes such values as truth, beauty, justice and so on. There is also another problem – what if the sum of happiness produces the greatest gain for two people out of 10, compared to a slightly smaller total sum divided equally among the 10 (Banks, 2006, p. 36)? The answer, for the utilitarians, is that the value of each person must count as one, and only one, so that the highly unequal outcome is excluded. In other words, if a lesser total amount of benefit is gained by the larger number of people then that should be seen as the better outcome. But, equally, one person cannot be irreparably harmed for the benefit of a group of others. Thus it may be reasonable to require those who earn more than others to contribute a greater amount of tax to a society, but only up to a point as it is not acceptable to impoverish one person because many others might gain from the redistribution of their wealth. From this, we have the principle of justice grounded in the recognition that each person ought to be able to assert her or his own view of what is good and right. (For the purpose of this discussion it is not necessary to go deeper into the finer points of the utilitarian approach, such as whether attention should focus on the outcomes of historical acts, the rules that ought to determine the best outcomes or the preferences of each person. The interested reader should consult MacIntyre, 1998, Rachels, 1998 or Freeman, 2000).

As Banks (2006, pp. 39 ff.) points out, in daily practice those in social work and human services, or indeed any other professional area, do not apply these approaches in pure form but work with an integration of these and other ideas at the points at which they can find agreement. For Banks, this bringing together of universal approaches forms a 'common morality' position (also see Beauchamp & Childress, 2009). This also resonates with Baldry's (2010) model of how human rights and social justice work together (see Chapter 2), even though one is based on deonto-logical assumptions and the other on a utilitarian approach. The extent to which these two approaches provide a universal ethical platform for social work and human services, to the exclusion of other ideas that might have something to offer practice, such as virtue ethics or the ethics of care, derives precisely from their capacity to be objective, separate from the values of any one individual person (compare Banks, 2006, with Webb, 2010). Thus they can be codified, inspected and appealed to, and form a quasi-legal set of rules. This may go some way to explaining what McBeath and Webb (2002, p. 1019) call 'the persistent drone' of deontology and utilitarianism, or a combination of them, in professional ethics.

Kantian deontology and utilitarianism, therefore, are universal ethical statements, and likewise the common morality that follows from integrating them. To recap, these approaches are based on premises about what it is to be human and can be brought to bear on practices that seek to address human need. Indeed, the notion of the free-dom of each individual to pursue her or his own view of what is good and right can be found in Maslow's universal concept of human need, derived from social psychol-ogy, which has been discussed above. The more recent theory of Doyal and Gough (1991) is more explicitly concerned with policy and politics. Their model consists of just two aspects, autonomy and health, which they do not place in a hierarchy. For

Doyal and Gough, both these needs must be satisfied in order for people to be able to engage with ordinary human life. They argue that these attributes are independent of each other but act together in the creation of possibilities for people to produce things (such as food, goods and services), to reproduce or to express a culture. Like Maslow, Doyal and Gough use data from different ethnicities and countries to develop their model, in order to be able to consider whether these factors apply to being human or to particular ideas about being human. To a much greater extent than Maslow, Doyal and Gough propose their theory of need as a statement of values: autonomy and health are conditions that people pursue precisely because they are necessary in order to live well as human beings. In these terms, the health needs of Maria and her family in the situation described at the beginning of this chapter are now met in her country of resettlement (although questions might be asked about mental health needs). However, their autonomy needs are not being met because the impact of trauma and the process of seeking asylum is limiting their capacity to live well, as this is understood either in their culture of origin or that of the place where they are resettled.

This notion of values in the analysis of human nature is grounded, at least in part, on the work of Sen (1985). Originally developed from economic theory, Sen's argument is directed to the question of poverty. Sen focuses on what he calls human 'capabilities' as the key to understanding what should be valued in life. In its simplest form, this approach considers poverty to be a question of what people can do with the things that they have rather than a simple numerical matter of how much wealth they possess. In other words, a person can be considered to be in poverty if they lack the capacity to engage in a reasonable life as this is understood within their own social context, separately from how financially wealthy they are. So, in the example of Maria's situation presented above, although she has sufficient material goods to live she still is not able to live well because she lacks ways of achieving other things that are important to her in her life, such as having good relationships with her husband and her children. In this, it would appear that Sen's approach largely agrees with that of Doyal and Gough, in that Maria and her family continue to be in need. These theories suggest that Maria requires assistance to develop her 'autonomy' or her 'capabilities' and that without these her life remains 'impoverished'.

Nussbaum (1998, 2000, 2006) argues that if understood broadly, human capabilities are not simply private preferences but can be seen as social attributes; moreover, these are 'cosmopolitan' in the universalist sense used by Kant. For Nussbaum, the universal aspect of these human characteristics is what is important, as she explicitly draws on a range of sources to develop her model, including Aristotle, Locke, Kant and Marx, whose ethical and political ideas are often considered as in conflict with each other. For this reason, it could be said that Nussbaum is also following the notion of 'common morality' (see above). Unlike Sen, who has refused to do so, Nussbaum has developed a list of the specific capabilities that she considers are universal. These, she states, are subject to empirical verification and indeed there has been a small degree of adaptation of the list over time. However, the list has remained substantially the same. The most developed statement of human capabilities is that which Nussbaum provided in her work on women and human development (2000) and this is summarized in Box 4.1. That this list is contained in Nussbaum's major work on women and gender in social development is significant, in that she developed this approach to universal values while engaged in cross-cultural dialogue and study: Nussbaum originates from New York, in the USA, and was working with women's groups in Kerala, in south-west India at the time she developed this framework.

Box 4.1 The 'central human capabilities' (from Nussbaum, 2000, pp. 78–80)

1. *Life.* Being able to live to the end of a human life of normal length; not dying prematurely or before one's life is so reduced as to be not worth living.
2. *Bodily health.* Being able to have good health, including reproductive health; to be adequately nourished; to have adequate shelter.
3. *Bodily integrity.* Being able to move freely from place to place; having one's bodily boundaries treated as sovereign, i.e. being able to be secure against assault, including sexual assault, child sexual abuse, and domestic violence; having opportunities for sexual satisfaction and for choice in matters of reproduction.
4. *Senses, imagination and thought.* Being able to use the senses, to imagine, think, and reason – and to do these things in a 'truly human way' [...] being able to search for the ultimate meaning in life in one's own way.
5. *Emotions.* Being able to have attachments to things and people outside ourselves; to love those who love and care for us, to grieve at their absence [and in general to experience the range of common human emotions, without having this capability impaired by fear, trauma, abuse, neglect and so on].
6. *Practical reason.* Being able to form a conception of the good and to engage in critical reflection about the planning of one's life. (This entails protection for the liberty of conscience.)
7. *Affiliation.* A. Being able to live with and toward others, to recognize and show concern for other human beings, to engage in various forms of social interaction; to be able to imagine the situation of another and to have compassion for that situation; to have the capability for both justice and friendship. [...] B. Having the social bases for self-respect and non-humiliation; being able to be treated as a dignified being whose worth is equal to that of others. This entails, at minimum, protections against discrimination on the basis of race, sex, sexual orientation, religion, caste, ethnicity, or national origin. In work, being able to work as a human being, exercising practical reason and being able and entering into meaningful relationships of mutual recognition with other workers.
8. *Other species.* Being able to live with concern for and in relation to animals, plants, and the world of nature.
9. *Play.* Being able to laugh, to play and to enjoy recreational activities.
10. *Control over one's environment.* A. Political. Being able to participate effectively in political choices that govern one's life; having the right of political participation, protections of free speech and association. B. Material. Being able to hold property (both land and moveable goods) [...] having property rights on an equal basis with others; having the right to seek employment on an equal basis with others; having the freedom from unwarranted search and seizure.

For Nussbaum, identifying shared concepts of what it is to live well is important for two main reasons. First, it emphasizes that human beings are inherently social – the capabilities cannot be achieved without addressing society 'as an organic whole' (2000, p. 74). Yet, second, at the same time it is necessary also to understand that 'the capabilities are sought for each and every person' (ibid.) and not primarily for collectivities (such as families, communities, nations or corporations). As Nussbaum strongly asserts, although these entities may be very important in achieving the capabilities, the goal must always be for them to be achieved by 'each and every person', treated as a person in her or his own right (ibid.). From this, it can be argued that Nussbaum's approach to the concept of capabilities resonates with the focus of social work and human services on 'the person in their social environment' (compare with Green & McDermott, 2010), as achieving the capabilities may require attention to personal and social rights and needs in conjunction with each other.

Nussbaum also notes that this approach has been criticized as encultured, namely as reflecting Western conceptions of what it is to live well. Her response is to note that, not only did she arrive at this understanding through her work with people of very different cultural backgrounds to her own, often in their contexts, but that it is deliberately written at a sufficient level of generality as to be shared across cultures while at the same time allowing for a rich variety in the detailed ways in which different people live and which they value (Nussbaum, 2000, p. 76). This critique from the position of 'cultural relativism' is the focus of the next chapter. Nussbaum's concept and her response to the critique are quite explicitly pluralist and this approach is then explored in greater depth in Chapter 6.

To take the example of Maria, who was introduced at the beginning of this chapter, it can be seen that her situation enables her to achieve some human capabilities, such as bodily health and bodily integrity. In a country of refuge she is now also in a place where she may be able to address some of the other aspects of living a human life more fully. However, at the same time, the impact of her flight from her home country apparently has been negative for her marriage and probably (it might be expected) for other family relationships, such as her loss of contact with those who were not able also to leave. She is also learning how to live in a new country with all that is involved in the process, including how she might begin even to think about planning for her future and that of her children. In different ways, therefore, the universal values that are embedded in these various approaches to human rights and human needs can be used to consider Maria's life and help those who are assisting her to examine the goals and methods of their work.

Universalism and culture: implications for practice and policy

Thinking about values and ethics concerns the goals (ends) and methods (means) of providing social work and human services and the connections between them. So in this way it has clear implications for policies, the structuring of institutions, and so on, and for all aspects of practice. However, while the significance of universal values such as human rights and social justice for policies and institutions may be easily grasped, the relevance for practice in the sense of the interaction between practitioners and service users may not always be so immediately apparent. Yet from the universal values perspective explained in the chapter it can be seen that human rights and questions of social justice are integrated in everyday experience and practice as well as in social policies or institutions, so both must be considered. As will be argued below, policy and practice are also always interconnected.

Colebatch (2009) points to the way in which policy must be considered as the interplay between objectives, strategies and customs, in which values provide both the background and the objective. Policy not only concerns how an issue or problem is analysed and ways of responding are formulated and organized: the definition of the issue or problem in the first place is the starting point for policy and this is inevitably value-laden. In this sense, social welfare institutions, governments and other actors in the social policy process inevitably are engaged with values as much as they are with matters of fact or technique. To some extent the values that underpin social policy are provided by the wider social context, but at the same time the various actors can also shape values through debate, through selecting particular issues to address or to ignore, through the use of objective data and so on. In a context in which universal values such as human rights and social justice are widely accepted these will set the stage for the policy process. In circumstances where these values are not widely accepted or not actually implemented, either other values will prevail or else social work and human services become engaged in advocating such a position. An example of the latter situation can be seen in the way in which anti-racism and anti-oppressive values were asserted and argued for by sections of social work and human services before they were seen more widely as core values for these professions (Dominelli, 2008; Clifford & Burke, 2009). As has been shown above, these developments are grounded in the universal values of human rights and social justice, with their emphasis on equity, respect and so on. From a universalist position, good social policy can be considered as that which clearly embodies these values.

Although some practitioners may find concepts such as human rights and social justice to be abstract and removed from their day-to-day work, thinking about them in terms of anti-racism, anti-oppressive practice and other more concrete expressions are more easily identifiable as relevant. Examples of this might include ensuring that practitioners are equipped in terms of skills and knowledge to work with people from cultures that are different to their own and that resources are distributed using criteria that are non-discriminatory. However, using universal values to think about other areas of practice is also important. For example, in work with older people, people with disabilities, people with mental health problems and other service users who are marginalized within the wider society, practitioners can encounter challenges to people's rights and inequities in responses from other professionals and agencies. One example that is often confronted in practice is the way in which adults with needs for care (because of old age, disability or mental health problems) can be assumed not to have the right to have their own view of their needs taken into account in decision making about services (for example, see Hugman, 2005, p. 157). So it should not be surprising that service users from among these groups can come to regard professionals as oppressive and people to be struggled against (Beresford, 2000, 2003; Postle & Beresford, 2007). Advocacy in support of these service users is part of direct practice, it is not only the concern of people engaged in policy and other less direct areas of work (see Sakamoto & Pitner, 2005). The values that underpin such work are universal, in that they form claims that rights apply to all people, irrespective of their health status or other aspects of their identity.

Clifford and Burke (2009, p. 7) argue that some of the reasons why practitioners may consider anti-oppressive values irrelevant or even harmful to specific practices are that they are poorly explained or taught, become co-opted, get overly simplified or are not subject to critical self-reflection. As Clifford and Burke note, criticizing anti-oppressive approaches, which are grounded in the universal values of human rights and social justice, on the basis of examples of poor practice is not a strong argument. In particular, they state that reflexivity and self-questioning is a core element of the anti-oppressive approach, precisely because it seeks to bring universal values to situations in which people of different backgrounds interact, whether this is difference of culture, 'race', socio-economic class, gender or other differences, in which ways of accessing social power are not equally distributed. As Dominelli (2008) points out, good practice, of which anti-racist and anti-oppressive approaches are a core part, requires the capacity to contextualize and think carefully about the nuances of any situation.

A further problem for anti-oppressive practice is that not everyone agrees that universal values are indeed universal. As has already been noted, it is argued by some critics that the concept of human rights is a 'Western' cultural construct and cannot be used in relation to people whose culture originates in other parts of the world (for example, see: Bell & Bauer, 1999). While the idea of social justice is less criticized in such overarching terms, in that as a broad idea it has a meaning in many cultures, what it might mean either more concretely in policy or in practice can also be regarded as encultured in the same way (Taylor, 1994, cited in Fraser, 2009). (Of course, the idea of social justice is criticized from within many cultures, for example on the grounds that it assumes that the goods that it requires to be redistributed are actually social – some critics consider that they can only be seen as properties or choices of individuals; for example, see: Grace, 1994). In social work and the human services such debates tend to focus more on the interpretation of universal values in working across cultures (Gray & Fook, 2004; Yip, 2004; Gray, 2005; Healy, 2007). That is, although the claim that there is a shared core of what it is to be human (Webster, 2002) is not rejected, it is argued that this is not helpfully addressed by taking a universal approach to values and ethics. Rather, this critical position emphasizes the differences between cultures as the point from which social work and human services should begin if the imposition of the most powerful perspectives on other groups is to be avoided. It is to that claim that the next chapter is addressed.

5   Cultural difference in values and ethics

The ethical challenge of cultural difference

Professional codes and statements on values and ethics commonly draw on universal approaches. Previous chapters have identified the major 'components' as the ethics of duty to principles based on human reason (deontology) and the ethics of consequences (especially utilitarianism). The ethics of character (virtue ethics), it has been noted, may also provide a basis for thinking about what it is to be a good social worker, child care worker, youth worker, community worker and so on, but is not as easily codified. It is also the case that these approaches are brought together so that elements of each inform everyday practice (see, for example: Beauchamp & Childress, 2009). Nevertheless, the key point is that all of these approaches are universal, both in their assumptions and in their implications. Yet at the same time, as noted in Chapter 1, ethics is the explicit deliberation about moral values and these cannot be assumed to be universal. As has already been shown through hypothetical case situations and other discussion, people differ in many ways in the things that they think are the most important aspects of life and, in some respects, they may disagree quite profoundly. So approaches to ethics that fail to take account of such differences could be seen as insufficient to deal with the complexities of social and cultural diversity.

It is on the challenge presented by diversity for social work and the human services that this book is focused. So in this chapter the discussion turns in greater detail to arguments for an explicit recognition of the way in which cultural differences ought to shape thinking about professional ethics. First, some detailed descriptions of practice are examined. Then, second, the chapter looks at key theoretical ideas about cultural difference and the notion of cultural 'relativity'. Third, in conclusion, it looks at the way in which arguments for cultural difference pose questions about whether social work and human services can be considered in global terms. This is of particular importance for several reasons: many of the societies in which social work and human services are professionalizing are or are becoming multicultural; the world is becoming increasingly 'globalized', with implications for the exchange of ideas and people in these professions; and, social work in particular but also other human service professions have developed international structures and practices over more than a century (Cox & Pawar, 2006; Lyons et al., 2006; Healy, 2008; Payne & Askeland, 2008).

Cultural difference and practice

In previous chapters various hypothetical practice situations have been presented, in each of which diversity of values are demonstrated. The questions explored in those examples can be broadened by asking what happens when practitioners are explicitly challenged by the idea of ethical relativism. This is shown in the following example.

> Joslyn is a community worker. Her family migrated from the Caribbean in the 1960s and she was born in an area of the city where she now lives and works in which the majority of the population is from a similar origin. Joslyn is very committed to using the knowledge and skills that she gained from her education and training to contribute to her neighbourhood, which faces a lot of issues in respect to poor quality public housing stock, limited employment opportunities (especially for younger people) and an increasing need for appropriate care for older people who are no longer able to cope on their own. Joslyn considers that part of her knowledge and skills that she can contribute come from her inside knowledge of the community, especially concerning values that are seen as a core aspect of culture. She has a good opinion of some of her colleagues who come from other cultural backgrounds, as do many community members, but Joslyn thinks that it is essential that as far as possible community workers should share the cultural background of those who they are assisting. At the same time, Joslyn recognizes that culture is not static and she considers herself to be connected both to the culture of her parents' origin and of the country where she was born and lives. For her, it is not a case of being stuck between 'cultures' but of being authentically 'black' in this context.

In another part of the country, a different situation is encountered by a social worker.

> Peter is a social worker in a children and family welfare agency. He is visiting a family in which a grandmother, Rose, is currently providing out-of-home care for two of her grandchildren, Skye (aged 9) and Justin (aged 14). The children's parents are separated and their mother, Rose's daughter, is unable to care for them because she is currently in a residential addictions programme while the children's father is in prison. The purpose of Peter's visit is to discuss with Rose the concerns that have been expressed by the school about her failing to ensure that the children attend school or to attend a meeting with teachers discuss some recent problems of the children's behaviour at school. Rose confronts Peter with the complaint that it is not possible to talk to him about these things: 'You're not from round here, so you don't understand us, you talk differently and you've been to college – so what use are you? What you think is right for children is not how we do things in this town.' Peter finds this ironic as he comes from a nearby town.

Joslyn's situation is easily recognized as one of 'culture' and its relationship to values. In contrast, it is likely that the situation faced by Peter would be widely understood as one of socio-economic class, which partly it is. However, Peter's situation concerns values and interpretations of those things that matter in understanding a good life, and in that sense, as discussed in Chapter 2, represents cultural difference as much as does Joslyn's. In particular, it can be noted that Rose is also understanding culture and values as related to regions within a country and other factors as well as to broader distinctions of 'race', ethnicity and nationality.

In different ways, both Joslyn and Rose are making claims that values differ between cultures and consequently community workers, social workers and others in the human services have to be able to relate closely to the culturally based values of those with whom they work. Joslyn is allowing that some workers can practise effectively in 'other' cultures (she has a good opinion of some of them) but in the context this seems to rest on their capacity to work within the values (and from this, the culture) of the community. This then raises questions about the professional values and ethics that such workers might be expected to hold and apply and whether these should be relative to any particular context. If so, does this mean that values and ethics are relative to each cultural context as opposed to being universal?

In a discussion of social work and human services provided to the traditional Muslim community in Toronto, in Canada, Azmi (1997) argues that cultural traditions are central to the consent of service users that is necessary for such services to be provided effectively. For Azmi, the problem of such situations is that they are not addressed by recognizing the indigenous values and practices regarding those things with which social work and human services are concerned. Azmi's critique is based on research which looked at 'individuals who were in some way involved in welfare response to wife abuse in the Muslim community' (1997, p. 103). This goes to the heart of the professionalization of these activities, which in traditional Muslim communities are actually regarded in an entirely different way, as matters of religion and family (pp. 104–105). In these circumstances, Azmi states that undertaking social work and human services in such communities is a form of 'ideological missionary work', in which modern secular values are imposed into a different value realm (p. 116). Seen in this way, Rose's reaction to Peter in the situation described above has many similarities – it is an invasion into her world of alien values (Hugman, 2005, pp. 130–132). Azmi's research also points to others within the Toronto Muslim communities whose position more closely resembles that of Joslyn, in that they accept the legitimacy of professionalized human services but consider that a worker has to be part of the distinctive cultural community to be able to practise effectively (1997, p. 106). In addition, there are yet others for whom the modernized professional understanding of human services is accepted, although Azmi suggests that these are either 'non-Muslim' or Muslims who are active in mainstream welfare institutions.

In these situations a range of positions on the relationship between culture and values are encountered. Although they differ between each other in the degree to which they accept the possibility of dialogue between value positions, they share a rejection of the idea that there are universal values that can apply in social work and human services. Furthermore, the basis for this rejection is that the things with which social work and human services are concerned are profoundly cultural and so the distinctions between cultures will necessarily generate diverse positions on values and ethics in different contexts.

The critique of a universal position on professional ethics and values

Midgley (1981) critiques the internationalization of social work as a 'professional imperialism'. That is, he argues that the types of theory and practice that have been developed in many parts of the word are mostly inappropriate because they are derived from the highly developed countries of Western Europe, North America and Australasia. Consequently the way in which social problems are understood and the practices and institutions being created to deal with these problems are based on cultural assumptions that have their origins in Europe. Both the goals of social work and human services and the means by which they are to be achieved thus are often highly unsuitable for the countries concerned. As argued elsewhere in this book, considerations of ends and means, as well as the connections between them, must be regarded as ethical and political as well as technical.

More recently, Yip (2004) has argued that this assumption of Western ideas and values as a universal norm has been restated in social work by the formulation of international statements on education and training and on ethics (IASSW/IFSW, 2004; IFSW/IASSW, 2004). Although contained within a wider criticism of a global view of social work as a profession, much of Yip's argument pivots on cultural difference in ethics (Yip, 2004, pp. 601 ff.). He concludes that the international organizations, although trying to find a way to recognize diversity, only manage to do this to a very limited extent. This Yip calls 'mild diversity', which he claims masks a highly Westernized view of social, political and religious values (p. 604). Moreover, he asserts that in many situations 'diversity' is actually a euphemism for ethnic minority values in multicultural societies where Western views predominate. Within that approach, Yip is suggesting, 'difference' is something allowed to minorities in a way that does not affect the 'real' values and ideas of the majority. In particular, Yip is concerned that as social work expands rapidly in Asia, its concepts and values should be related to cultures informed by Buddhism, Confucianism, Hinduism, Islam and Taoism. To demonstrate this point, Yip focuses on Chinese cultural values, with particular reference to their Confucian foundations. These values are compared with Western values as often being entirely opposed in their meaning and implications. This comparison is summarized in Table 5.1.

In each case, Yip argues, the international documents on social work make assumptions about the nature of social work, its goals and methods, that are based on the Western cultural values as listed here. This is seen to be unacceptable both because it represents the continuation of an implicit imperialism (which, ironically, is contrary to such values) and also in that it leads to ineffective practice in non-Western contexts.

To illustrate this point, Yip provides short case vignettes taken from work with domestic violence, workplace injury, child abuse (with aspects of alcohol misuse), residential aged-care and mental health. A central theme in each of these vignettes is

Table 5.1 Chinese and Western cultural values compared

Chinese cultural values	Western cultural values
responsibility	rights
social norms	equality
family	individual
stability	change
relation	empowerment

Source: gleaned from Yip, 2004.

the way in which people holding traditional Chinese values, whether living in Hong Kong or Australia, were helped more effectively by attention to their values. The practices that are described are then explained as contrary to Western professional values. Most especially, the refusal of the individuals concerned to assert rights claims in a legalistic way is a common thread. Yet the outcomes described are often very similar to those that might be aimed for by a human rights perspective, as in the examples of a woman subject to domestic violence leaving her husband and a man addressing his alcohol dependence and stopping abuse of his children. Yip's point is that these were achieved through practices based on the traditional Chinese values listed in Table 5.1 and not on the assertion of individualistic rights claims (as his particular focus of Western values). For example, the woman leaving her violent husband did so on the grounds of her responsibility to protect her daughter, rather than her rights to self-protection; the man addressing abuse of his children and alcohol dependence by seeking assistance to change his behaviour did so because the intervention focused on the background values of family, social norms, responsibility, stability and relationships which he understood and accepted.

There are also criticisms from African perspectives that the normative positions embedded in 'international' professional ethics and values are framed from a Western perspective (Osei-Hwedie, 1993; Graham, 2002; Osei-Hwedie *et al.*, 2006). For Osei-Hwedie and his colleagues the growth of social work in Botswana only became relevant to the needs of the country when it responded to the cultural, social and political realities. This required a shift from a dominant concern with individual welfare and institutional care to social and community development. Within this, the values of Botswana's ethnic groups (which they describe as broadly similar, see Osei-Hwedie *et al.*, 2006, p. 571) are shown to be focused on community relationships and people being empowered to contribute to the society, as opposed to the 'imported' values of autonomy, self-determination and so on. This echoes points made previously by Silavwe (1995) writing from Zambia. Particular reference is made by these and other African social workers to principles of *ubuntu* (connectedness, identity in relationship to community), *ipelegeng* (fulfilling social responsibilities) and *ma'at* (acting justly, with wisdom) (also see Graham, 2002). Each of these ways of understanding what is good is distinctively African and does not sit comfortably with the more individualized concepts that tend to define professional ethics derived from deontology or utilitarianism. In particular, Graham emphasizes that *ma'at* is not only a description of a state or abstract principle, but rather an action that ought to be accomplished: it demands that a person should 'speak truth, do justice and walk each day in the path of rightness' (Graham, 2002, p. 80). Identifying the core values in these ideas as the integration of the individual with community and of action with thought can, therefore, be seen as challenging the dominance of Western values.

This critique has been developed more broadly by Gray and Fook (2004), Noble (2004) and Gray (2005) in discussion of ways in which ethics and values can be considered across cultural diverse situations. While their overall concern lies beyond ethics as such, encompassing all aspects of social work and human services, these analyses build on the concept of 'professional imperialism' as a continuing problem. In particular, Gray and Fook (2004) and Noble (2004) identify claims to universal values as a central feature of 'professional imperialism'. Gray and Fook (2004) argue that in order to overcome this tendency it is necessary to consider approaches to understanding all aspects of social work and human services, beginning with what is considered normative in each localized context. In other words, the process of making connections or investigating what is shared ought to commence from a recognition of the diversity between different situations, rather than by looking to find ways of grounding universal values through seeking those points of apparent commonality in ways that do not challenge the assumptions of the universal position. By focusing attention on that which is common as the basis for international ethical discussion, these critics argue that difference is obscured and does not get addressed. Clifford and Burke (2009, pp. 35–38) summarize this view as a call for a reflexive approach in which those who hold dominant value positions can consider the position of others and listen to what is being said.

So far, it is possible to reframe these arguments in terms of 'good practice'. When a social worker or counsellor does not provide appropriate support for a woman who experiences violence from her husband, or any professional fails to take action to ensure a thorough investigation of the suggestion that a child is at risk of serious harm, these could be regarded as instances of poor practice in many different cultural situations. Indeed, when the examples provided by Yip are considered, in those situations where people are at risk interventions are aimed at addressing this, while in other cases the prevailing approach is to work with the service users' views about desired outcomes. In the broadest sense this way of thinking could be said to be closely related to the ('Western') principle of self-determination, which in some discussions of social work and human services has at times been accorded the status of a primary value. As Nimmagadda and Cowger (1999) note, this principle, as usually presented may not be appropriate for all Asian cultural contexts. What is at issue is the detail of *how* the professional should respond and this also demonstrates underlying professional values. In Nimmagadda and Cowger's study of social work and human services in India, giving direct advice and reinforcing traditional roles, relationships and duties were explicitly used as techniques, based on a straightforward acceptance that, as professionals, social workers and others in the human services have authority and with that an obligation to use it deliberately. In a different example, in Vietnam human services workers might deliberately withhold negative information where it is thought that this would undermine the hopefulness on the part of a service user and their family that is considered necessary to promote coping or healing, but some self-direction is also valued (Nguyen Thi Thai Lan, 2011).

Attention to cultural relativity of values has two major areas: cross-cultural practice, in which the practitioner and the service user are from different cultural backgrounds; and variations between encultured ways of thinking about practice, in situations where ideas are exchanged between cultures, as in the international context at conferences or in professional literatures. In both areas there is a need to be sensitive to cultural expressions of values and the implications that these may have for different conceptions of good practice. This point might then lead to the conclusion that there are no such things as single global constructions of social work, youth work, community work or any other human services practice, because each ought to be seen as unique to the cultural context in which it is practised. In other words, that what social work, youth work, community work and so on actually *are* is different relative to culture.

Cultural and ethical relativism: the debate

Moral philosophers are concerned with two distinct forms of relativism: cultural and ethical (Williams, 1972, p. 34). There is a common aspect to these concepts, in that they are both based on the idea that normative values will reasonably differ between individuals and groups. The difference between these two concepts can be understood by looking at the question of 'relative to what?'

First, cultural relativism can be said to be the position that has so far informed the discussion of this chapter. That is, it holds that values and other aspects of ethics may reasonably differ between cultures. Indeed, philosophers such as Williams (1972, 1981), along with anthropologists such as Westermark (1932) and Benedict (2005 [1934]), argue that all such differences between cultures should be regarded in relative terms. All cultural groups have a history and traditions that inform the normative basis of what it is to be an appropriate member of the group. So what is regarded as good or right in one culture may be regarded neutrally or negatively in another. For example, it might be seen that one culture regards individual freedom as the most important value against which everything is judged, while in another culture adherence to shared community norms is considered the benchmark of what is good and right. From this position, what is considered right and wrong in one culture may be reasonably regarded differently in another. Because the points of reference are grounded in those cultures there is no basis for making judgements between them, so it is important that the values of each culture be taken as the basis of ethical judgement in that context. So, in this view, when someone such as Joslyn in the situation described above encounters colleagues from other cultural backgrounds and whose values differ because of this, it is simply a fact that must be accommodated, through asking simply whether the other person is appropriate to work with this particular community or not.

Second, ethical relativism holds that the claims of different ethical approaches cannot be evaluated against a single notion of truth (Williams, 1972; compare with

Hinman, 2008). It does this at both the meta-ethical level (theories of ethics) and normative ethics level (concepts of good/bad and right/wrong). At the more general level, ethical relativism argues that there is no basis for making judgements between value positions. From this, normative ethical relativism proceeds to argue that claims about particular values, for example that it is wrong to lie, have no universal applicability because their truth depends on the relative context in which they are asserted. Ethical relativism can be argued from a range of different standpoints. For example, the truth of a value claim can rest on circumstance, or the goals that one is trying to pursue, or personal preference. Indeed, it is logical that no one of these positions should be seen as determining, as they are themselves relative to the standpoint of the value holder. So whereas cultural relativism assumes a degree of consistency within a culture or society, ethical relativism allows for differences between members of a society.

Some arguments for cultural relativism are not extended to ethical relativism. For example, Williams (1972, 1981) argues that ethical differences between people who share a cultural background are best understood as a matter of choosing between workable alternative courses of action. This is quite different to cultural diversity, because it holds that within a particular culture it is possible through reflection and debate to consider who is right and who is wrong. Cultural diversity, for Williams, is the main arena of relativism because it generates competing belief systems that may or may not have the capacity to talk to each other. So for Williams while cultural relativism is plausible, ethical relativism is not (in fact he is quite dismissive of it, see: 1972 p. 34). More recently philosophers such as Hinman (2008) have rephrased this distinction. Hinman distinguishes between 'descriptive' relativism, which can be understood as the statement as a matter of fact that people in different cultures have different moral beliefs, and 'normative' relativism, in which any moral belief can only be valid in the particular culture from which it originates (2008, p. 34). For Hinman, the implications of these ideas when combined can lead ultimately to the notion that moral values can only be relative to each individual. Such a position is known as 'ethical subjectivism'. It holds that each person's subjective view of the world is relevant for them and there is no basis for comparison or dialogue other than as a matter of fact. When ethical relativism is encountered within a culture (because, being within the culture it cannot be cultural relativism) then this is the logical conclusion. Hinman concludes that in the modern world this position 'is often conveyed through a shrug of the shoulders and a "whatever"' (p. 37).

In some ways the situation of Peter and Rose, above, is also one of relativism, except it is not a matter of 'whatever' but rather that Rose considers Peter's values to be inappropriate. The phrase she is most likely to use is to say that Peter is 'wrong'. The assertions Rose makes can be summarized in the form 'you are not like us', which is a claim that encompasses the things of culture, including how a person thinks and feels, how they talk and so on. So this also seems to be a form of cultural relativity and not simply subjective difference. However, because Peter and Rose would in other respects be regarded as of the same culture this interaction might also be considered as an example of critical debate about what should be considered right and wrong.

Certainly Rose seems to see it that way. For someone in social work and the human services these distinctions are important, because the professional task must be accomplished through interpersonal communication and without an effective basis for this the task appears futile.

It is also the case that if Rose is correct and that having a high level of education is part of what creates such difference, then by definition it is unlikely that any other social worker would meet her expectation of 'being like us'. What is encompassed by professional education means that even if a practitioner's origins were in the exact same locality (recall that Peter comes from the same part of the country), the very act of undertaking professional education would create a very strong probability that the social worker would have engaged in the sort of critical reflection that Williams (1985) argues is the basis for changing our own ethical positions. Williams (1972, p. 35) also holds that Rose's claim to a cultural distinction is dubious, because the boundaries around cultures are not necessarily that solid (compare with Hinman, 2008, p. 36). For example, it may be that Peter was born and grew up locally but his values have developed away from those that Rose regards as culturally 'local' precisely because he has undertaken higher education and professional training. This is what Azmi (1997) is indicating as a potential barrier to the idea of people from 'within' a culture becoming professionalized so that service delivery becomes more 'appropriate'. For Azmi, it is the very idea of professional services responding to such issues (domestic violence, substitute child care and so on) as opposed to these being the province of religious leaders or other designated community members that is regarded as culturally alien, along with the laws and policies on which professional practices are based.

The idea of cultural competence

The position described above for Joslyn may also be expected to be quite similar to that for Peter in some respects. Although she is a member of the cultural community in which she works, she also has undertaken professional education and training. Yet from these accounts it would appear that she is accepted by the community as working in a way that does not confront wider values. This raises two possibilities. One is that the tasks that each role has to perform might be regarded differently. The role of the community worker is likely to involve engaging with those problems and issues that members of the community agree should be dealt with (Butcher *et al.*, 2007). Its understanding of the cause of problems and issues and its focus of change primarily lie outside the community. In contrast, the role of the social worker includes acting as a representative of the state to supervise social welfare arrangements as well as to focus on the person and the resolution of relationship problems and issues, as the cause (at least potentially and partially) as well as the target for change.

The other possibility is that Joslyn has developed greater 'cultural competence' (as have some of her colleagues) whereas Peter has not. This concept refers to a way of looking at work between cultural positions in which the professional approaches the interaction as a matter of knowing both about the other culture and also that person's own culture, so that inappropriate impositions of values do not occur. As Dean (2001) observes, the aim of this approach is that the professional will then be able to focus on the values, needs and other aspects of the service user (whether an individual, family, group or community) in the service user's own terms. As Dean describes it, this approach has developed from knowing 'about' 'other' cultures in a not very sophisticated form of anthropology, to a more considered recognition that the practitioner also has a culture and has to be critically aware of this (2001, pp. 625–626). Central to this approach is a shift from an externalized understanding of culture as something possessed by others to an intersubjective view of culture as something that is part of the world-view of every person. ('Intersubjective' here means that what is being sought is an understanding of the values of both people in the interaction and of the way that they either support or confront each other.)

The way in which this conviction about an intersubjective understanding of values may be achieved is through reflecting on one's own ideas and beliefs and comparing these with others (Williams, 1985). For Williams the practice of reflection is the key to a relative understanding of ethics and values. Through such a process, it is argued, it becomes possible to recognize that one's own values do not have any particular universal objectivity (that is, they are not factually 'true' in the sense that laws of physics can be shown to be objective). Then, in turn, it is possible to grasp the positions of others. To do so does not require that one's own value judgements have to be abandoned, because the positions of others are not objective either (Altham, 1995). What is required in this relativistic view of ethics and values is that each person develop confidence in her or his own position through constant reflection on what seems best, what most fits the world as it appears to the person making the evaluation.

Such an approach has become influential in social work and human services through the notion of 'reflexivity' (Gould, 1996; Taylor & White, 2001; Fook, 2002; Taylor & White, 2006). While in these professions this concept has been derived largely from thinking about knowledge and research methods (what is known in philosophy as 'epistemology') rather than ethics, it offers social work and the human services a way of thinking that is broad and can encompass ethics and values. In this way it connects with the ethics of philosophers such as Williams. For Fook, 'reflexivity [refers to] a *stance* of being able to locate oneself in the picture' (2002, p. 43, emphasis original). In other words, it requires a degree of self-consciousness in which the position from which one is looking at the world and the cultural differences between oneself and others is seen as relational. The 'otherness of the other' is understood only by being aware that one's own cultural position is also perceived as 'other' by that person. Most importantly that which is most significantly different between the practitioner and the other is the values that each holds and their cultural basis. Thus, Taylor and White (2006, p. 948) argue, reflexivity requires recognition by the practitioner that in human services all practice decisions and actions concern values as well as technicalities. Reflexivity in this sense is a search for wisdom in dealing with uncertainty, not for a certainty that removes considerations of value.

In the context of thinking about ethics and values in cross-cultural practice, reflexivity offers a method of achieving what Dean (2001) describes as 'not knowing' (as the alternative to cross-cultural competence as a form of objective knowledge). Similarly, Gray (2005) use the term 'humility'. What Dean and Gray mean here is that the practitioner ought to start from the position that she or he does not have the depth of understanding of the ideas and beliefs of the service user and so should not introduce and impose her or his own attitudes and values but listen and learn from the service user. There are some echoes here of Socrates' ancient claim that the beginning of all wisdom is 'knowing what one does not know' (MacIntyre, 1998, p. 20). In the situation of Joslyn and her colleagues in the situation described earlier in this chapter, whose work is considered to be relevant by the community, it is likely that either they hold values that are congruent with those of the community or else they have developed a way of working that embodies this openness to learning from the community.

Peter, however, is in a different situation. The functions of his role appear to preclude him from achieving the same type of acceptance because he has goals that are set from outside the working relationship with Rose and her family. Although he may seek to express these in ways that he thinks might make it easier for Rose to understand, if she regards these as an 'alien imposition' then it could reasonably be asked what opportunity Peter has for being able to work across this cultural difference. One answer is to say that he does not have to, he simply is required to state the law and any relevant policy and to discuss their implications with Rose. There is a statutory requirement in the country in question that all children must attend school until the age of 17 and if they do not do so parents or guardians are held accountable; it would not be appropriate for Peter to act as if this was not the case. This has similarities with the situation faced by the practitioners working with the Botshoma family in the example of different cultural views about physical chastisement of children discussed in Chapter 2, who are expected to work within the child risk and protection laws and policies. It may also be argued that how Peter communicates the requirements of law and policy with Rose and other family members is an important element of good practice in this situation. Part of the professional role in such a situation is also to make sure that people understand the laws and policies, to give them the opportunity to express their thoughts and feelings about their circumstances and to consider options. In the end, Rose's options do not include both conforming to the law and allowing the children not to go to school and Peter must find a way of communicating this to her. Graham's (2002), Yip's (2004) and others' ideas about working in different ways in different settings may be useful to Peter in thinking about how he could work across this particular relative gap between world-views. The discussion returns to the implications of these issues in Chapter 9.

Ethical relativism appeals to social workers, community workers, youth workers and others in the human services because of its assumptions that each person is entitled to their own value position (Sercombe, 2010, pp. 39–40). As Sercombe notes, it avoids the possibility of arrogance that is implied by an absolute universal position and validates the service user, in situations where service users are often devalued.

There is a similarity here with Gray's (2005) notion of 'humility' in working between cultures. Relativism is the opposite of saying 'I know that my views on this are correct so if you think differently then you are simply wrong'. In occupations that are seeking to enable disadvantaged or troubled people to find their own voice, including their moral voice, such an orientation is congruent with the wider purposes of professional practice (compare with Koehn, 1994). Associated with this are the goals of tolerance and acceptance that reflect the aim of helping others to achieve empowerment in their lives.

'And yet ...'

Having reviewed the arguments for relativism and considered some of its implications, this discussion is left with a problem that is inconvenient, at least for an uncritically relativistic position. This problem can be stated in a number of different ways, but at its centre is the philosophical question of whether tolerance and acceptance of positions other than one's own ought to have no limit. As Williams (a philosopher often credited as a major proponent of ethical relativism) observes, such a position is self-contradictorily absolute (1972, p. 35). In other words, it attaches a non-relative value to relativistic goals of tolerance and acceptance, so that these values become absolute. At the extreme the internal logic of the argument becomes one of saying 'there cannot be any all-embracing universal position', which is itself a universal and all-embracing statement.

For Williams (1972, 1981, 1985), therefore, the answer is to seek a more subtle way of thinking about the way in which moral claims can be made and the relationships between the people who are making them. Such a position can also be seen in the anthropology of Benedict, who is also sometimes credited with the promotion of cultural relativism regarding morality, in her clear ethical attacks on racism as well as her use of evaluative terminology such as 'fiction' or 'excessive' to describe certain complex marriage customs where these appear positively harmful to individuals (2005 [1934], p. 33).

Similar practical limitations to relativism can also be seen in the debates of social work and human services. One of the clearest examples of this can be seen in the way in which neither Azmi (1997) nor Yip (2004) can be taken to be implying that interpersonal violence within families is acceptable (they are not even saying that it is at least morally neutral). In fact, both these arguments are framed around the idea that such things as domestic violence and the abuse of children are wrong. In Azmi's (1997) discussion, the question of culture concerns who should intervene and not whether intervention would be appropriate. This is a dispute over the way in which domestic violence is understood, the moral constructions of its causes and its resolution. For Azmi, the traditional Muslim community of Toronto should have the capacity to assert that these things are the province of religious rather than secular ideas, values and practices. Yip's (2004) position is somewhat different, in that he is writing as a social worker for whom the idea of intervention to assist a person facing such problems is framed in professional terms. What is at issue for Yip is the very particular understanding of cultural values and the way in which these are used to orient professional practice. These two arguments share a moral concern with the phenomena of family violence as 'bad' and a criticism that the construction of professional social work as they observe it is founded on Western values. Where they part company is on who should respond and how (compare with Hugman, 2008). Of course, cultural relativism easily allows for such differences, treating them as facts rather than as right or wrong. However, the moral basis of these arguments raises the question of the extent to which difference precludes the possibility of ethical agreement across cultures.

In the context of considerations of African values, having asserted the primacy of principles such as *ubuntu, ipelegeng* and *ma'at*, with their emphasis of community over individualism, Graham (2002), Osei-Hwedie (2003) and Osei-Hwedie *et al.* (2006) then also weave claims to human rights and social justice into the moral fabric. The way in which these concepts are understood and used in these discussions has great similarity to the way in which it would be used in Europe, North America or Australasia. As with Yip, a more complex picture emerges of the claims to cultural relativity lying as much in the context and detail as it does about the more general idea of professional social work and human services. Moreover, although Graham (2002, p. 64) makes a strong argument that speaking of large cultural groupings makes comparative sense, what she calls an 'underlying philosophical unity', both Graham and others also note differences *within* as well as between such groupings. Thus, while at one level it makes good sense to speak of 'African', 'Asian' or 'Western' values, this should not be done without also recognizing that the unity of these constructions becomes evident only when they are regarded as different relative to each other. In the era of European colonialism this has meant that the 'West' (that is, Western Europe) has been the focal point of comparisons, as shown by the way both the African and Asian perspectives above are argued against Western values. But from other standpoints there are clear relative variations *within* each of these broad cultural constructions. The different parts of each broadly understood cultural region may also perceive themselves to be distinctive, such as in the variations between northern and southern Europe in expressions of the form a good family should take. While this does not in itself challenge the claims of relativism, it does raise some questions about how much an uncritically relativistic position can provide the basis for a shared professional ethics, whether at national or international levels.

From this, we can see that the possibility of interconnections between different cultural positions on ethics and values both within and between countries is crucial for social work and the human services. As has been noted above, and in previous chapters, one aspect of this process, especially for social work, has been its development as an international profession. The underlying implication of one reading of Gray and Fook (2004), Noble (2004) and Gray (2005) is that an international concept of such professions is not plausible. However, it is a conclusion that they are reluctant to reach. Along with Midgley (1981), Osei-Hwedie (1993), Nimmagadda and Cowger (1999), Graham (2002), Osei-Hwedie *et al.* (2006) and others, what is being sought is a discourse on values and ethics that addresses cultural relativity in the same way that discussions of indigenization consider the moulding of skills and knowledge to any particular social and cultural context.

While some of the debates discussed here stem from challenges to this, at the same time this does not prevent people in many countries from seeking to adapt and use these professional theories and skills to address the issues and problems that they see in their own societies. For this reason, although it is very important that such adaptation and development should be appropriate to each context, recognition of commonalities that enable conversations to take place between people from different cultural backgrounds is also crucial if such international dialogue is to be able to take place. But more than that, the occurrence of such conversations over a very long period of time leading to some shared perspectives on matters such as social justice, for example, adds to reasonable doubt about whether cultural relativism of moral values is the best way to understand the differences that culture introduces to professional thought. Quite simply, in practice, social workers, youth workers, community workers and others regularly go well beyond Hinman's 'shrug of the shoulders and a "whatever"' (see above). Graham (2002, p. 97) concludes her analysis of an African perspective on ethics and values with the suggestion that 'a diversified philosophical base [could encourage] social workers to view their mission in broader terms'. This aspiration implies that through embracing diversity, and especially for practitioners from the historically dominant West in learning from other parts of the world (compare with: Gray, 2005; Hugman, 2010), it may be possible to seek unity *in* diversity. Yet if it is to do this there must be some ground on which values and principles can be examined, carefully considered and either accepted or set aside. Unless this can be achieved, simply tolerating the differences between cultures can only be achievable through the separation of communities or the abandonment of any claims to internationally recognizable shared professional identities.

Sercombe summarizes this problem clearly. Having argued that 'the standard position in most of the human services is relativism' (2010, p. 39), he then proceeds to question whether culture can be used as a moral defence for certain acts, such as rape, murder and so on. This leads him to the conclusion that '[t]o say that a belief or practice is cultural doesn't mean that it isn't wrong' (p. 40). The challenge then is to be able to say what we can agree between different cultural positions can be said to be right or wrong. This echoes Hinman's (2008) observation that in the last two hundred years many societies have changed their practices in relation to things such as the punishment of people who commit crimes (death sentences for theft have been replaced with imprisonment or fines), slavery has been abolished, and so on. It is not just that 'we now have different standards' but that these changes came from the asserting that the new standards are 'better' (Hinman, 2008, p. 48). The values that some relativist arguments have criticized as 'Western' can thus themselves be seen as development away from the more traditional values of Western cultures (which in many ways had closer resemblances to some aspects of those asserted by the critics as Asian or African) (compare with Hugman, 2008). Moreover, the changes in these values were fuelled as much by moral argument as by other factors. Recognizing this capacity for cultures to change, sometimes quite rapidly, identifies another problem that relativism has to grapple with, namely that it tends to treat culture as fixed and immune from criticism.

So where does this leave the social worker, community worker, youth worker and others in human services who wish to pursue values of acceptance and cultural humility? A third possibility in ethics, which seeks to avoid the extremes of universalism and relativism, developed in the twentieth century. This is the approach of ethical, or value pluralism (Berlin, 1969, 1992; Hinman, 2008). This position has had relatively little attention in social work and the human services, but offers ways to think around the problems that have been identified here. So it is to this task that the next chapter turns.

6 Pluralism and ethics in social work and human services

What is ethical pluralism?

In the previous two chapters the competing positions of universalism and cultural relativism have each been discussed. Both influence debates in professional ethics. Yet if taken simply as mutually exclusive stances, it may appear as if what ought to follow is either to join the battle on one side or the other, or to stand back and observe the arguments as an interested bystander in describing them and commenting on their contributions to thinking about ethics. However, these are not the only choices. A third possibility is opened up by considering that the claims established by both universalism and cultural relativism require attention, but without any one position trumping all others. This approach is called 'pluralism' (sometimes 'value pluralism' or 'ethical pluralism') (Berlin, 1969, 1992; Kekes, 1993; Hinman, 2008). Pluralism can be summarized as the position that argues morality cannot be seen as 'singular' or 'unitary' but that '[t]here are many truths that are sometimes partial and some-times conflicting' (Hinman, 2008, p. 49).

This chapter begins by explaining ethical pluralism and then looks at the implications this approach has for thinking about social work and the human services. It examines pluralism both in practice and in thinking about wider questions such as codes of ethics and the use of social power. In particular, the challenge of this approach is how to identify those values that are shared and how to resolve disagreements about those that are not. This chapter examines pluralism as distinct from both universalism and relativism and considers the way it addresses the weaknesses of these other two ethical approaches.

Pluralism accepts that the values people hold may be incompatible and so in conflict with each other (Berlin, 1969, 1992). An example of this that is relevant for social work and the human services is the possible incompatibilities of 'equality' and 'freedom'. Both these values may be held to be primary in the modern world and yet there will be situations, possibly many, in which the achievement of one appears to reduce the possibility of the other. For instance, if varying life opportunities result in some people being very wealthy while others live in poverty this could be regarded as bad; however, if the only way of alleviating poverty is to compel the wealthy to give up some of the goods they have acquired then this can be seen as a constraint on freedom and that may be seen as bad as well. In this way it can be seen that across a society, or between cultures, it can reasonably be expected that there may be such conflicts arising from the incompatibility of values. Rawls' (1972) formulation of a theory of justice is perhaps the best known attempt to resolve this incompatibility through a balance between the two values, in that it seeks to reconcile the ideas of freedom and equity (as fairness). However, it is not universally accepted precisely because people differ in the ways in which they think freedom and equity can or should be pursued (see summary by Grace, 1994).

Furthermore, pluralism also argues that some values simply cannot be compared (Berlin, 1992; Kekes, 1993; Gray, 1996; Chang, 1997). This concept is referred to either as 'incomparability' or as 'incommensurability'. To give a very simple illustration, people might value the beauty of the natural world and also value the family as a social institution. Such values may be held equally strongly as very important. Moreover, both these values may be held at the same time without any conflict. It is not the case that the more of one that a person enjoys, the less of the other will be achievable. So any attempt to identify a hierarchy between such values simply makes no sense.

Yet Kekes (1993, p. 22) also points out that values may be both incompatible and incommensurable. That is, it may be both impossible to achieve all shared values at the same time and impossible to compare them in such a way that an order of priorities can be established. While many conflicts can be sorted out by developing ranking systems, this too is unlikely to resolve the problem across a society: such 'rankings are reasonable only in particular situations because they depend on the variable and individual conceptions of a good life held by the participating agents' (Kekes, 1993, p. 23). So while it may be possible for an individual to achieve a workable balance between competing values, even to vary the balance between different types of situation, the wider this approach is taken the more problematic it becomes. So, to use another of Kekes' examples, the values of justice and friendship can pose exactly this type of problem. An individual may find acceptable ways of achieving balance between the problem for justice of partiality that arises when actions favour one's friends, and the problem for friendship of impartiality when choices seem to be disloyal. However, for a whole society such attempts are likely to prove contentious for some if not for many. Thus what can appear in one society to be 'nepotism' (bad) can in another society be held to be the 'honouring of social obligations' (good) (compare with Nagel, 1979). The instances in previous chapters concerning family relationships and responsibilities (discipline of children, care of elders) are connected to this point in different ways; this aspect will be discussed more fully below in relation to the ethics of care.

Ethical theories and approaches can also be regarded as in conflict in this way and, at times, as not capable of being compared (Hinman, 2008). In this understanding, focusing on duty of respect to the inherent moral character of humanity (deontology), on consequences of choices (consequentialism) or on the moral character of human actors (virtue) poses different types of question in each case. There are instances where there may be no conflict, for example one in which the question about poverty that is posed by the notion of equity can be approached deontologically, consequentially or in terms of virtue. The deontologist might argue that the acceptability of poverty is not a maxim that can be universalized, the consequentialist argue that the sum of human well-being is diminished by the existence of poverty and the virtue ethicist argue that failing to alleviate poverty stems from a lack of compassion or the 'vice' of indifference to the suffering of others. In this sense they can agree on the implications of their different approaches without having to be in agreement on the way such conclusions are reached. However, in many situations it is equally if not more likely that there will be some disagreement between ethical approaches about choices for action that arise from the values that are embodied in these approaches. So, if the consequentialist argues that the alleviation of poverty requires a limit to the amount of wealth that any one individual can possess (Singer, 2002; Solas, 2008), the deontologist might begin to have concerns about the resulting ethical cost of limiting human will and responsibility (Nozick, 1974; Grace, 1994), while the virtue ethicist approaches this from a different angle and asks about the balance of competing qualities in the actors involved (Webb, 2010). In such a situation consequentialism and deontology seem incompatible, while virtue ethics appears incommensurable with the other two approaches. As the basis for decisions about practice and policy there is thus no single reasonable way of stating a hierarchy but there remains a plurality of possibilities, each of which may have something reasonable to say about the issue or problem. This may go some way to explaining the relatively limited impact of virtue ethics on some formal ethical debates within professions, especially as reflected in codes of ethics.

Following Berlin, Kekes and others, Hinman (2008) is careful to explain that pluralism is not a form of relativism in disguise. He argues that it should be seen as distinct from claims that there is no such thing as 'moral truth' (which is technically called 'nihilism') or that such truth just depends on one's own point of view ('subjectivism'). What is important for Hinman is to look at ethical questions from the perspective that moral disagreement is inevitable and, furthermore, this can be a strength rather than a weakness in solving ethical problems. The advantages of such a position are that it does not depend on different positions being compatible but rather that they can often provide checks and balances against each other in the questions they raise (Hinman, 2008, pp. 53–54). Moreover, pluralism encourages the sort of 'humility' that was briefly mentioned in the previous chapter (compare with Gray, 2005). This involves listening to others and considering possibilities for agreement before disagreeing and asserting one's own prior position. As far as possible, pluralism promotes the goal of living with difference while recognizing that there are times when decisions have to be made that favour one or another perspective (what Nagel, 1979, calls 'points of singularity').

So, pluralism recognizes that there are plausible cultural differences in values and that these lead to questions about the ways in which context shapes the ethical understanding that people have of the world. At the same time it seeks to promote conversations between positions, which requires that people find ways of being able to talk to each other. This encourages the discovery of those values, both moral and non-moral, that can be shared between cultural settings. As will be discussed in more detail below, this hope of conversation carries risks. When that which separates people is too great or the likelihood of compromise is low (because one or more of the participants in the conversation has the clear intention only of winning the argument, for example, rather than listening to other points of view) then a conclusion can be very difficult if not impossible to reach (Hinman, 2008, p. 54; also see Habermas, 1990; Rorty, 1999).

To assist in thinking about how a pluralist position can be approached, Kekes (1993, pp. 38 ff.) makes a helpful distinction between 'primary' and 'secondary' values. The difference between these two orders of value can be seen as follows. Primary values may be seen as those that can be widely agreed between competing cultural positions as providing the minimum necessary conditions for the achievement of what can be agreed as a decent human life. Kekes' starting point (1993, p. 39) is that water, food, shelter and general bodily health seem to be shared across humanity as a species. Beyond this it may also be possible to identify some psychological and sociological factors that tend to be characteristics of a decent human life across different cultures, at least seen in general terms, such as being safe, experiencing emotions and motivations or being part of social groupings (p. 40). This list has very strong similarities with the human needs identified by Maslow (1954; see Chapter 4). Gewirth (1978) makes a similar point in his argument that the two basic human needs, in this sense, are health and freedom (the discussion returns below to these factors). The distinctive contribution of these approaches to the possibility of widely shared ideas about what people value is that the lists start by focusing on non-moral objectives. In this sense, non-moral goods can be seen as those things that are naturally occurring and affect the person making the evaluation, whereas moral goods derive from human action and affect others with whom the person interacts (Kekes, 1993, p. 45). Primary values are 'thin' concepts of 'the good', to paraphrase Walzer (1994). In this context, the idea of 'thin' refers to the way in which such lists are as small or narrow as possible, demanding as little as possible of what human beings might value while still describing a decent life, to the point where agreement is most likely. This is a quality of argument that philosophers call 'parsimonious'. Such an approach does not necessarily reduce the range of reasonable options for acting: it is from a parsimonious view of primary values that a pluralist such as Hinman wishes to speak about the limits of tolerance and acceptance and 'standing up against evil' (2008, p. 55). Even Rorty (1999), for whom even Hinman's position is too universally inclined, actually favours democracy and egalitarianism as basic values, in such a way that although totalitarian and hierarchical systems can be understood as rational they can still be opposed because it can be argued that they do not provide the best way to meet a minimum shared view of a 'good human life'.

Secondary values, in contrast, are those that give substance to the primary values in any given context. These are Walzer's (1994) 'thick' concepts of what is good. They consist again of both moral and non-moral values, but here a greater degree of concrete detail is found. These are statements concerning the form in which appropriate nutrition is achieved, of how relationships should be conducted, who counts as 'family', of the choices people should make in acting towards each other in private and in public, and so on (compare with Kekes, 1993, pp. 42–43). For example, while all human beings need nutrition, the form that this should take to achieve a decent life (should it be noodle soup, chicken vindaloo, nachos or fish and chips – or, indeed whether one should be able to choose between all of these in a food-hall) will depend on a persons' cultural background.

Value pluralism and practice

The things that concern social workers and others in the human services can be seen in the same way. Close human relationships, what Kekes (1993, p. 41) calls 'goods of intimacy', may form primary values, but the exact shape and structures of families vary according to culture. For example, the roles that are ascribed to particular bio-logical relationships are not the same in all societies and the experience of family life seen as good in one culture may be regarded as inappropriate or even as unacceptable in another. Similarly, as has been noted at several points in previous chapters, appro-priate means of rearing children, including discipline, or of providing care for depend-ent adults vary between contexts; even what clothing is regarded as decent in public settings can be a source of difference and disagreement. The challenge for social work and the human services is to engage with this distinction between primary and sec-ondary values in such a way that the sometimes inevitable conflicts between second-ary values are resolvable in some way.

The following situation illustrates the way in which these questions can be faced in practice. While this example is distinctively Australian (and has strong parallels in other 'settler' societies, such as Aotearoa-New Zealand, Canada and the USA), there are also some broader comparisons that can be drawn with those countries that have communities defined by immigration from former colonies (mostly the European countries) (compare Green & Baldry, 2008, with Clifford & Burke, 2009). In par-ticular, this illustration draws attention to possible conflicts between primary and secondary values that are experienced in terms of cultural difference, which have a long and complicated history.

> Tanya is a mother of two daughters, one aged 5 years and the other 6 months. Her partner Dave, the girls' father, is currently in prison for several offences that include assaulting Tanya. Both Tanya and Dave are Aboriginal Australians and members of families in the communities that are the traditional owners of the land in the city where the live. Child protection caseworkers from the state gov-ernment child and family services agency were involved in an assessment of the family's situation just before Dave was arrested. While relieved at not experienc-ing violence, Tanya is still finding it difficult to cope with the children and misses Dave. She has assistance from various members of her wider family that includes members of three generations. Both her mother and her grandmother were 'taken into care' (under previous policies, as part of what is now known as the 'Stolen Generations'). So Tanya and her family are reluctant to seek help from human

services agencies, although they need assistance with housing and social security. Tanya is pleased to find that a local community organization has been given some funding by the state government to provide support to Aboriginal mothers and so asks for their help. However, Beth, the Aboriginal support worker who is also from the local community, has concerns that even though Tanya is getting child care help from her family there are still some risks to the safety of the children, particularly the baby, in the form of neglect. Although she is very committed to understanding the situation of her own people in terms of human rights and social justice, the question facing Beth is whether to work for longer with the family as culture suggests, to further support their strengths, or to interpret her responsibilities as a professional worker as requiring that she should notify the state child protection agency.

The question of the 'Stolen Generations', in which Aboriginal children were removed from their families into state care on grounds of 'race' rather than welfare, has been a significant contribution to the ongoing Aboriginal experience of colonization (Briskman, 2007; Green & Baldry, 2008). Under this policy children were separated from their families, placed in institutions and thus also prevented from learning about and being able to grow up in the practice of their culture. The same pattern of negative effects of institutional care, and the same prevalence of abuses that have been noted in other contexts was experienced (compare with McLeod, 1999). However, in addition there have been the effects on a whole culture of the systematic removal of large proportions of several generations. Simply arguing that decisions about child protection (or, indeed, any other matter of social welfare) are now made on the same grounds for all sections of the society does not address the extent to which the situations faced by Aboriginal families stem from the history of colonization, the systematic breaking up of families and communities and the impact of these processes on current generations. This example portrays a family in crisis and risks playing into stereotypes, but it also gives an account of issues faced disproportionately by Indigenous people not only in Australia but also elsewhere (Blackstock, 2004; Weaver, 2004; Green & Baldry, 2008).

Making practice choices about right actions in this situation can be seen either as a struggle to find the 'correct', or perhaps the 'best', ethical approach – or it can be regarded in terms of value pluralism. If human services professions do not pursue the idea of there being one single 'right' way to act in any given situation, however, understanding the implications of a pluralist approach for decisions making and dialogue within and between professions needs to be addressed. At the outset one particular point needs to be restated. As has been made clear in previous chapters, this is not an argument that law or policy can be ignored. In all the states and territories of Australia there are child protection laws that constitute a framework of requirements for various professions. Any professional decisions must be seen in relationship to these laws and policies. The notion that practitioners choose between competing values is not an argument for a free-for-all or that anything goes. What Beth, in the above practice example, is faced with is the judgement of knowing 'when different is just different and when it is wrong' (to paraphrase Donaldson, 1996, in Healy, 2007, p. 13; compare with Hinman, 2008, p. 55).

As a starting point, as an Aboriginal woman Beth knows that there is nothing in Aboriginal culture that finds the ill-treatment or neglect of children to be morally acceptable. Although the detail of what counts as appropriate care of children varies between cultures, it is very hard to find historical examples where there are not expectations that children will be cared for. (The point about the effectively universal normative valuing of children is discussed in Chapter 2.) Certainly for Aboriginal Australians it is the case that the care of children is a strong cultural value. Indeed, the title of the report of the Northern Territory Board of Inquiry into the Protection of Aboriginal Children from Sexual Abuse, *Little Children Are Sacred* (BIPACSA, 2007) is translated from a Yolngu saying which reflects the centrality of children to such a culture.

In pluralist terms any questions about the relationship between Aboriginal people and human services systems is not about the primary values concerning children; their safety and security are seen as important by everyone. Much of what occurs in the way in which Aboriginal people are misapprehended by professionals and service systems lies in what a pluralist view would regard as secondary values, which shape the way in which primary values are achieved. Factors such as who counts as family, or how competing claims of family and community are balanced with other obligations (such as in the priority of ceremonial responsibilities), can be causes of conflict between Aboriginal and non-Aboriginal Australians. There are strong parallels here with the debates already noted in the previous chapter concerning Muslim communities in Canada and the application of Western social work with Chinese people in Hong Kong and Australia (Azmi, 1997; Yip, 2004). In each of these situations social workers, community workers and other human service professionals face a refusal to engage with practices that are seen to reflect Western values. However, in each of these situations the overall objectives were for women to be protected from family violence, children to be cared for appropriately and so on. These are aspects of living well that can be readily agreed across cultural boundaries. For the pluralist, in these situations finding such agreement at the level of primary values helps in then thinking beyond the tangible cultural differences. Indeed, such differences are not only to be accepted but also to be positively affirmed as much as is possible. Here the pluralist position recognizes that debates about *who* should act, *how* they should act and even *why* actions should be pursued are inevitable. Furthermore, it is not only a fact that such debates occur but it should be regarded as good that there is at least the possibility of disagreement about such matters.

It should be emphasized that it is the *possibility* of disagreement that is important in pluralism, not that conflict is to be celebrated simply for its own sake. Disagreement both forces people to rethink the expression of their values and may, if handled positively, lead to acceptable accommodations of difference. So the ethical challenge faced by Beth in the situation described above should not be seen in stark terms as just that of notifying the statutory child protection authority of concerns or taking the responsibility for this decision on her own as if she is not part of a wider network of relationships, both community and professional. It is an example of the realities faced by practitioners in many contexts that value differences have to be negotiated and if forced create or sustain relationships of oppression. (The discussion returns below to the issue of power in social relationships that this raises.) Given the statutory nature of many human service practices, in child protection, mental health, criminal justice, social security and so on, accepting that there may be incompatibility and even incommensurability of values involved is not a problem 'to be overcome' but one with which it is necessary for practitioners to learn to work (Healy, 2005).

Professional ethics and value pluralism

In the most comprehensive internationally comparative study of social work professional ethics that has been undertaken, Banks (2006) looks at a form of pluralism in her discussion of 'common morality' in professional ethics. This idea is taken from bioethics, specifically the arguments of Beauchamp and Childress (2009; compare with Banks, 2006, pp. 39 ff., who cites an earlier edition of this work), in whose view the health professions have developed an applied ethics that brings together elements of deontology, utilitarianism and virtue ethics. Instead of looking at values, Beauchamp and Childress focus on four principles a synthesis of which forms the basis of ethics in the biomedical field: autonomy; beneficence; non-maleficence; justice. These can be summarized in the following way. Autonomy here concerns respect for the capacities of people to make choices based on their own values. Beneficence reflects the goal of maximizing benefits and as far as possible minimizing risks, while non-maleficence (also known as 'non-malfeasance') has a long history in the form of 'seeking to do no harm'. Justice, in this model, focuses specifically on fairness in the distribution of benefits and risks. Having reviewed this approach, Banks (2006, pp. 42 ff.) then compares it with the main influences in social work ethics as deriving from Kantian deontology, utilitarianism and what she calls 'radical' principles. Drawing on Beauchamp and Childress' concept of 'common morality', Banks argues that these three approaches are synthesized in social work and each make a contribution to the profession's ethics. Elsewhere Banks also applies the same analysis to human services, community work, health professions and youth work (Banks, 2004; Butcher *et al.*, 2007; Banks & Gallagher, 2009; Banks, 2010). Deontology and utilitarianism have been explained elsewhere in this book; by 'radical' here Banks is referring to the concept that what it is to be human is socially structured and so it is necessary to consider ethics and values from a social perspective rather than relying on individualist liberal ideas that underpin other modern approaches to ethics. In some respects, in Banks' discussion utilitarianism and radicalism have strong similarities, for example in their emphasis on justice and utility in their deliberations. At the same time, deontology and radical ethics share a concern with human rights, while deontology and utilitarianism have a common respect for the value of people as individuals. Thus the three approaches stand as a 'tripod' of principles on which contemporary social work and human services practices are located.

Drawing on other writers, such as Clark (2000), Banks (2006, p. 47) notes that at the more applied level of ethical codes, ethical terminology and focus within social work and human services can vary. At times concepts such as 'citizenship' (seen as the right to receive services) may be identified, in other places 'promotion of welfare' is seen as a central principle, and at other times there is a concern with 'service' (including integrity, competence and the like). (It is important to recognize that service here has to be seen as an ethical orientation on the part of professionals, even as a verb in the sense of being 'what professionals do', and 'not a noun, not something we deliver' [Sercombe, 2010, p. 12].) From this variation in terminology Banks (2006, p. 47) concludes that 'there is not one commonly agreed and coherent set of principles' for social work and human services. Yet there are also enough common ideas for codes of ethics around the world to reflect similar concerns and for the international bodies to have a statement on ethics, which itself takes the common morality position Banks describes, and which is agreed to by professionals from many countries in the context of, and despite, robust debate.

This analysis leads Banks (2006, p. 66) to argue that the professional ethics of social work and human services is pluralist. To consider how this affects the ways in which practitioners might engage with ethics, Banks looks at the work of Nagel (1979), in which he argues that morality in everyday life consists of making practical judgements between values. For Nagel (1979, pp. 129–130), the primary values in question are: obligations (to family, friends or colleagues for example); rights and responsibilities arising from them; the benefits or harm caused by one's actions ('utility'); the intrinsic meaning of something (such as artistic or scientific endeavour – Nagel calls this 'perfectionist ends'); and one's own life projects. The challenge of the way in which each of these places demands on each person is that they may often be in conflict, but:

> [t]he unavailability of a single, reductive method or a clear set of priorities for settling them does not remove the necessity of making decisions in each case. When faced with conflicting and incommensurable claims we still have to do something – even if it is to do nothing.
>
> (Nagel, 1979, p. 130)

According to Nagel (p. 135), this situation leads to a 'fragmentation' in our understanding of values, meaning that there is not one right way to think about ethical problems or to resolve ethical challenges. Consequently, we require the development of practical wisdom in order to make the difficult decisions that have to be made, using a concept first developed by the ancient Greeks such as Socrates and Aristotle. Banks (2006, p. 68) makes the point that in discussions of ethics, rational principles tend to be used because this provides a framework for reflection. However, in practice other factors, such as emotional responses, relationships between people, assessment of specific situations and so on all play a part in the exercise of practical wisdom (compare with Webb, 2010). This faculty also has similarities with the notion of reflexivity that was discussed in the previous chapter.

Other analyses of professional ethics reach similar conclusions. For example, Clark (2000) identifies the need for the tensions between different approaches to be understood and considered, especially between deontology and consequential arguments. Bowles *et al.* (2006, pp. 82–84) agree with Banks that although this is a necessary process, such tensions are to be seen not only as inevitable but also as a positive contribution to the implementation of ethics. Furthermore, they argue that the objective fact that ethics in the professions is necessarily plural is in itself one of the reasons why professionalism is important and that the roles of professionals cannot be reduced to prescriptive sets of organizational procedures (see Chapter 3). So, for Bowles *et al.* (pp. 115–116), the debates and disagreements between members of the same professions on the prioritization of human rights or social justice, in situations where they are in conflict, is precisely where the means to understand and to develop the moral base of these professions comes from. From this, Bowles *et al.* appear to agree implicitly with Nagel's notion of practical wisdom which they perceive as a skill, something that can be developed over time and which can be understood as '360-degree assessment' (2006, p. 207). By this, they mean that all aspects of a situation are considered and decision making leading to action, including not doing anything, follow from this process. There are clear parallels here with the notion of reflexivity discussed above, in that both objective and subjective factors are taken into consideration, including those concerning the practitioner's own self. However, Bowles *et al.* are offering a practice model, what might be termed an applied ethics approach, which they suggest is different to other 'decision making models' in that it is cyclical rather than linear. This means that it is possible to enter the process at different points: the practitioner can begin by reflecting critically on their goals, or the demands of policy, or the values that different people involved bring to the situation. There is also no fixed point of decision, but this too must be reached by consideration. Indeed, in some ways, such a model can be seen as a continual process for the critically reflective practitioner that will continue across a range of situations.

To return to the illustrative example above of Beth with Tanya and her family, it might be expected that as an experienced practitioner Beth has developed a sense of being able to find balances between competing values, those of culture, her profession and the state law. She knows who in each of these domains is likely to agree with her and support her decision or to disagree with her; she may well have discussed this with them in reaching her decision on what action to take. She will take into account her knowledge of the family and of the wider community, of their strengths and capacities, and of other resources that are available to them. This includes professional ethics and values, but these are not to be understood as prescriptive in the same way that an agency procedure manual might be. A code of ethics still requires practice wisdom so that it is used well, which in turn involves a capacity to engage with culture in professional action.

So for Beth, in the challenges she faces in providing community support to Aboriginal mothers, the concept of pluralism in professional ethics does not mean that she is unable to reach a conclusion and act. Rather, it suggests that she can draw on a range of ideas and values to make a decision about the best course of action in this situation at this time, while also allowing her the scope to continue to think about and develop her practice through integrating ethical considerations with other aspects such as technique, law and policy, her organizational setting and so on.

Addressing power – pluralism, human rights and social justice

One of the central concerns of professions such as social work, youth work, community work and other human service practices, is that of communities or families and individuals who are in some way disadvantaged, marginalized or excluded from the mainstream of their societies. On a global scale this includes a concern with questions of social and community development and needs faced by particular countries or even regions. As England (1983, p. 13) remarks about social work, it exists not to help people who have problems but for people 'who cannot cope with their problems unaided'. Butcher *et al.* (2007) make similar points concerning community development. Likewise, for Sercombe (2010, pp. 22–24) the main focus of youth work is with those who experience, or are at risk of, disadvantage, marginalization and exclusion on grounds of their age (compare with Banks, 2010). So the relationship between human services and those who use them tends, with almost no exceptions, to establish relationships of social power in which the authority, influence and capacity to act of professionals is greater than that of service users (Hugman, 1991). Such power is grounded in the formal roles that professionals occupy, which are often mandated by the state or other large institutions, as well as knowledge and skill. (Indeed, as may seem obvious, without these capacities service users would most likely look elsewhere for assistance where they have the choice.) Moreover, the problems and needs faced by service users are likely to have dimensions that can be understood in terms of social divisions or stratifications, such as sex and gender, sexuality, 'race' and ethnicity, disability (physical or intellectual) or age (at both ends of the life course, that is childhood and youth as well as old age). For this reason these professions are often responding to the impacts of sexism and patriarchy, heterosexism, racism, disablism and ageism. If a pluralist approach to ethics is to have meaning in these professions it has to be able to provide a basis for considering these aspects of the social world.

A major criticism of value or ethical pluralism is that it is seen to fail in providing a basis for drawing a moral line on questions of social power, especially of its abuse (whether implicit or explicit). Of course, this is the criticism from universal or monistic perspectives concerning issues such as human rights and social justice. For example, from these positions pluralism is seen to fail in providing a firm enough foundation to be able to say that human rights apply equally to all people in all situations. In contrast, the relativist position considers pluralism to leave open the back door for a covert form of universalism to return by stealth. From this perspective, pluralism is criticized as seeking to find shared values that apply to all people. There is, perhaps, more strength to the second than to the first criticism. As already noted above, proponents of pluralism find no problem in taking clear stances on moral questions. However, this does not mean that they prescribe ways of achieving primary values. Rather, pluralism seeks to extend as far as possible the opportunities for people to pursue those things that they regard as valuable in life, which differ greatly between individuals and communities.

For example, Kekes (1993) writes about the 'need for limits'. For him, looking at this question begins with the central moral goal of the possibility of a decent human life. So Kekes has no hesitation in describing 'slavery, female circumcision, racism, blood feuds, foot-binding, child prostitution, political corruption, torture, arbitrary imprisonment, the mutilation of criminals, and other similar notorious and regrettably widespread practices' as 'evil' (1993, p. 119). Likewise, Hinman (2008, p. 55) states:

> It is important, at least in cases of egregious moral wrongdoing, to speak out against offenses wherever they occur, whether in one's own or another culture. This is of particular importance because often the most outrageous wrongdoing is directed against the powerless of the world: children, women, and minorities (whether these are racial, ethnic or religious minorities). An account of morality that provides no moral foundation for opposing such wrongdoing falls far short of the mark.

So, although Kekes' list of evils looks somewhat more arbitrary than Hinman's, they share the view that setting limits is both possible and desirable. Moreover, there is a commonality to the ideas that underpin these statements, which might provide a clue to the values that they could agree as primary. These can be seen as 'health' and 'freedom' (compare with Gewirth, 1978). In other words, for the achievement of human lives in which people have the capacities that are required to make the sort of judgements inferred by both Kekes and Hinman, it is necessary that people have both sufficient personal health (physical, psychological, emotional and spiritual) and freedom as individuals and as members of communities (compare with Nussbaum, 2000). At the same time, the detailed form that ways of achieving and expressing these things will take is regarded by pluralism as contingent on the different secondary values that people hold. Examples include the way in which people relate with others in their communities, the form of family and other intimate relationships, and so on. (This point is pursued in greater depth in Chapter 9.)

Dominelli's critique of racism in social work and the human services (originally published in 1988) addresses this complexity by considering the phenomenon of racism and its impact on professional practice as having individual, cultural and social structural dimensions (Dominelli, 2008). That is, it is both possible and necessary to identify racism in the beliefs and actions of individuals, in culturally shared values and in the operation of organizations and social systems together and at the same time. The ethical implications of this analysis must therefore draw on a plurality of critical values concerning the way in which anti-racist practice is constructed.

First, deontology highlights the way in which racism operates through the dehumanization of 'others', in that a failure to give the same value to each person irrespective of their ethnicity demonstrates a disregard for the acceptance of moral duty towards shared humanity. Yet at the same time, a simplistic use of deontological theory can lead to a 'one size fits all' way of thinking, in which reasonable cultural differences are ignored. This in turn can lead to an expectation that ethnic minorities will assimilate to majority cultures, so that social work and human service practices are exactly the same in all situations (Dominelli, 2008, pp. 72 ff.). In addition, as Clifford and Burke note (2009, p.70), this approach can effectively ignore the structured inequality in capacity to access rights or to develop the capacity to make decisions and so obscure those inequalities and oppressions.

Second, a utilitarian approach provides the basis for focusing on the outcomes of practice. Questions that Dominelli raises about the inadequacies of human services provision for members of ethnic minority communities (as well as, often, for majority community members) can partly be answered by looking at the balance of outcomes. If the cumulative costs of inadequate human services are taken into account, the 'economies' achieved in the present are likely to produce greater costs in the future (compare Dominelli, 2008, pp. 117–118 with Gauntlett et al., 2000). However, a simplistic approach to utilitarian principles often results in inadequate provision for ethnic minorities, because the idea of 'scale' is attached to 'economies' and there is insufficient appropriate differentiation (Dominelli, 2008, p. 124).

Third, therefore, the radical perspective offers the opportunity to consider social structures as forming and sustaining implicit as well as explicit racism in social work and human services. This understanding identifies the grounding of racism in the lack of justice in meeting needs, which are defined in terms of the collective outcomes for members of communities. Redistribution of goods and the empowerment of people as members of communities are the goals that this approach identifies. Thus, in response to a recognition of racism, the appropriate needs of members of ethnic minorities should be attended to by a specific focus on challenges to structural inequalities (compare with Banks, 2006, p. 43). However, a simplistic 'radical' perspective can obscure the individuality of people: as Dominelli makes clear (2008, p. 74) shared culture does not necessarily mean complete agreement on values.

In this way, a thorough critique of racism in social work and human services points to a pluralist understanding of values and ethics. In a more recent detailed discussion of practice implications of anti-oppressive ethics and values Clifford and Burke (2009) implicitly argue for a pluralist approach. They consider deontological, utilitarian and virtue ethics, as well as the ethics of care and the recognition of a structural analysis that points to multiple (intersecting) social divisions (racism, patriarchy, disablism, heterosexism, ageism) (compare with Hugman, 2005). Although they do not refer explicitly to pluralism as such, their argument is that each of these perspectives has something important to say to practitioners, while requiring careful judgement to be made in any given situation. Likewise, McAuliffe and Chenoweth (2008) argue for a similarly integrated model of ethical reflection. Social structural understanding of human needs and issues faced by service users and human services professionals are a central factor in these discussion, particularly as this avoids the individualization of ethical responsibility that can tend, unhelpfully, to suggest that each practitioner acts on their own.

The analyses of Banks (2006), Dominelli (2008), McAuliffe and Chenoweth (2008) and Clifford and Burke (2009) all demonstrate the importance of a pluralistic approach to ethics in social work and human services. It is important to see these various arguments as expressions of pluralism, even where the term is not used explicitly. In particular, while each discussion looks at the plausibility of a range of values and ethical responses, none of them conclude by arguing for a relativism that leaves the practitioner unable to find ways of making judgements. As was noted above from Kekes (1993) and Hinman (2008), setting moral limits is both necessary and reasonable. As Dominelli puts it in her argument for the need to be ethically sensitive as a first step to anti-racist practice (2008, p. 74):

> Becoming ethnically sensitive is not about tolerating dehumanizing or violent behaviour as 'culturally appropriate' in unfamiliar cultures. The challenge for practitioners is to investigate a situation, reflect critically upon what is needed and intervene without disparaging service users, and draw upon a wide range of resources in doing so. ... Saying 'no' should not be confused as racism.

Underlying this argument is an acknowledgement that any culture contains disagreements and that values are always contested, whether the culture in question forms the majority or is in a minority situation (Dominelli, 2008, p. 74). It is also important to recognize that 'setting moral limits' is something that occurs in majority cultures as a consequence of critique and debate. An example of this is the shift in European cultures around issues such as family violence and child abuse, where criticism and debate within majority cultures has produced significant change, even though it can be argued that much more needs to be done to protect women and children, and some men, from violence that is buttressed by patriarchal values (Hugman, 2008).

Ethical pluralism for social work and the human services

There are two particular problems for a pluralist ethics arising from the structural analysis of disadvantage and oppression. The first of these is the potential for a pluralist view of freedom to leave unchallenged such inequalities, precisely because it does not provide an unequivocal voice against such matters as being morally unacceptable. This issue is addressed in greater detail in Chapter 8; however, at this point it is useful to note that this argument is effectively addressed in social work and the human services, as Dominelli's (2008) statement above demonstrates. For now, it can be observed that the uses of pluralism as an ethical theory to favour an individualistic view of liberty or freedom do not prevent the development of other understandings that hold the notion of plurality of values while also engaging with the struggle to identify the 'moral limits of tolerance'. It is, rather, that critical thinking about these ideas can help in the construction of positive arguments for practices and policies that seek to create circumstances in which more people may achieve the sort of freedom envisaged by Berlin (1969), Kekes (1993), Rorty (1999) and others. Making connections between anti-racism, anti-sexism and other oppositional strategies does not have to deny freedom of thought and action for anyone; it would be a self-defeating argument if it did. Rather, Dominelli's careful but critical analysis of racism shows that a structural understanding does not have to be in conflict with the recognition that there are differences within as well as between cultures and communities.

A pluralist approach also offers an alternative view on the problem, as it is often seen, of having to choose 'the lesser of two evils' that occurs in many situations (Banks, 2006, p. 25). The notions of incompatibility and incommensurability suggest that value conflict is inevitable (Gray, 1996; Hinman, 2008). So this suggests that the necessity of choice without an obvious single rational basis for decision is sometimes inevitable (Nagel, 1979). How this is to be handled by practitioners is addressed in slightly different ways in various discussions although there is a common thread. Banks (2006, p. 25) suggests that careful thought that considers the known facts of a situation, the technical and policy issues and the ethical aspects before reaching a decision on 'the least worst outcome' will tend to produce practice integrity. Bowles *et al.* (2006, p. 42) describe a process of 'bounded ethical decision-making' in which making judgements that are 'as good as possible' should be the aim of the practitioner. Similarly, Sercombe (2010, p. 71) argues that it is sometimes necessary to seek a workable compromise, as any practitioner will be surrounded by people who may or may not agree with all of her or his core values. Others, such as Hugman (2005) and Clifford and Burke (2009) present detailed discussions of the range of contemporary ethical theories that offer something to a pluralistic professional ethics. These are not arguments for a relativistic 'whatever' (Hinman, 2008, p. 45). Rather they are calls for social workers and others in the human services to seek to become 'morally active practitioners' (Husband, 1995). They are also quite explicitly not calls for any practitioner to give up the values that they hold to be important. Instead, these arguments point to the need for practitioners to be more aware of the basis for the values that they do hold, so that such values may be shared with others in a reasoned way, even when they are communicated with passion and conviction. This in turn requires attention to some possible ideas for thinking about the practice of pluralism in professional ethics and values.

To summarize these various arguments, Table 6.1 presents key ideas that provide a basis for undertaking this process. These are suggested here as an aid to critical thought and not as a prescription or a 'how to' list of instructions, which in an argument for a pluralistic perspective would be ironic at the very least. Nor necessarily should these ideas be read as a suggestion of virtues, although they are to some extent personal qualities that can be developed by practice; rather they are 'ideas for practice'.

In the situation facing the Aboriginal community support worker, Beth (see above), being able to think about professional ethics in this way, within the context of her identity as an Aboriginal woman and her role as a human service professional, the complexities of the values that contribute to understanding good practice need to be emphasized. As an Aboriginal worker, Beth is very conscious of her own positioning and she wishes that, although some of her mainstream colleagues show the same ability to be reflexive, others also could do so. This would create a better opportunity for more open dialogue about the difficulty of working with conflicting values, including

Table 6.1 Key ideas in pluralist ethical practice in social work and human services

Key idea	Practice focus	Aim in pluralist ethics
Clarity	Explicit attention to ethics as part of professional skill and knowledge	Awareness of the values that are being pursued and what they contribute to understanding 'good practice' in a given situation
Persistence	Accepting that achievement of values is not always quick and easy	The capacity to pursue values over time, so that a 'win or lose' is avoided
Humility	Accepting that others may have reasonable but different points of view	Incorporating the idea that plurality of values occurs between people and groups as well as within them; 'different' does not have to mean 'wrong'
Reflexivity	Recognizing that values come from one's own positioning	The capacity to reflect on one's own contribution to shaping ethical considerations; listening to others while maintaining a sense of one's own ethical self

those within the local Aboriginal community as well as between the community and the mainstream. Such a dialogue could overcome the way that internal community differences are often currently used against the interests of community members. However, Beth has also learned that if she and those colleagues who she sees as supportive are to be a positive influence on the values of the agency and the surrounding society then giving up is not the best option.

This chapter has examined value or ethical pluralism as a distinctly different approach to those of universalism and relativism. It has argued that this way of looking at ethics in social work and the human services has the potential to address the limitations of the other two approaches. Having established this perspective as distinct, in the next two chapters the discussion explores in greater depth two areas of human life and thought that are central to concepts of 'the good' and which have both contributed to the development of social work and the human services, namely religion and spirituality and politics. So, Chapter 7 considers the implications of a pluralist approach for re-examining the relationship between religion and spirituality and professional values and ethics. Chapter 8 then picks up some threads that have begun in this chapter and looks in more detail at politics and political morality in relation to these professions.

7 Religion, spirituality, values and ethics

Implications for social work and human services

Religion and spirituality in social work and human services

Religion and spirituality can be considered as inter-related concepts, which concern phenomena that are experienced across human cultures. Using a common distinction, religion can be seen as 'an organized, structured set of beliefs and practices shared by a defined community that are related to spirituality' and spirituality can be understood as 'the search for meaning, purpose, and morally fulfilling relation with self, other people, the encompassing universe, and ultimate reality, however a person understands it' (Furman *et al.*, 2004, p. 772; compare with Burton & Bosek, 2000, p. 98). Religion and spirituality therefore form an important part of the value frame of reference for individuals and communities. Yet, through the twentieth century, the place of religion and spirituality in social work and human services became ambiguous if not completely marginal. This may seem surprising, as the nineteenth-century origins of social work, youth work and community work in Western countries were often grounded in the application of religious concerns to the social problems and issues of the day (Forsythe, 1995; Canda & Furman, 1999; Bowpitt, 1998; Payne, 2005; Sercombe, 2010). Payne (2005), in particular, charts the gradual emergence of professional social work and other human service practices out of the secularization of Christian charitable action over a period from the seventeenth to the late nineteenth centuries, notably in Western Europe and its (then) colonies. He also notes the extent to which, in other parts of the world, religions other than Christianity can be regarded as having produced the sorts of practices that can be regarded as proto-professional social work and human services (Payne, 2005, p. 19; compare with Faherty, 2006, and Graham & Shier, 2009). Writers from Eastern traditions such as Buddhism also find it possible to see such connections, as do those from Indigenous and African spiritual traditions (Yellow Bird, 1999; Graham, 2002; Leung *et al.*, 2009). Nevertheless, by the end of the twentieth century mainstream discussions and theorizing of professional knowledge, skills and values had tended either to become silent on matters or religion and spirituality or to confine such questions to a specialist concern with specific cultures, usually those considered as 'minorities' (Hodge & Limb, 2010). This is an approach to religion and spirituality that can be described as 'secular public theology' (McFayden, 2002) or 'practical atheism' (Whiting, 2008).

(This latter concept arises specifically from a consideration of social work and human services.) However, in practice it may even lead to the deliberate ignoring of religion and spirituality, with this exclusion seen as an ethical choice (Burton & Bosek, 2000).

There are two possible explanations for the obscuring of religion and spirituality in these fields. The first of these is the rapid secularization of modern society, especially through the twentieth century. Indeed, to describe societies as secular and modern may even seem to be a tautology. In particular, in Western countries, the public role of religion has changed through the processes of the Reformation, the Enlightenment and the Industrial Revolution. Increasingly diverse views on religious beliefs and practices mean that it is not possible to assume that all of the people who otherwise share a culture will view particular religious ideas as providing a unifying expression of commonly held social values. What has come often to be shared between those holding quite divergent views about religion and spirituality is a commitment to scientific rationality, not only in science itself but also in the way in which such things as social issues and problems were to be addressed (Whiting, 2008). Within this process, ethics can also be regarded as having been 'secularized'. Examples include Kant's 'reworking' of the older 'golden rule' (versions of which exist in many of the world religions) into the categorical imperative (Banks, 2006, p. 29) and the arguments for atheism of Nietzsche in what may be seen as a form of ethical egoism (Hinman, 2008, p. 117) and Marx in a particular consequentialist form of social justice (Reisch, 2002, p. 345). Some of these approaches, such as that of Kant, are effectively neutral about religion as such, while others, such as Nietzsche and Marx are explicitly negative. As O'Hagan notes (2001, p. 142), this period of European intellectual history is marked by growing mockery and hostility towards religion. This view is shared by many present members of the human services professions, often amplified by phenomena such as the abuse of children by clergy and the apparent reluctance of institutional churches to address this scandal, as well as more generally by fundamentalism, cults, sexism and other values that some interpretations of religion appear to support (O'Hagan, 2001, pp. 139–144).

As Graham and Shier note (2009, p. 217) some commentators describe these professions as effectively taking over from religion in the fields of social welfare, personal well-being and so on. While the argument that social work and human services have 'taken over' religious functions is a contentious one, there is nevertheless an historical coincidence of secularization and professionalization in these fields. For many practitioners, whether or not they hold religious beliefs themselves, and in many texts about these fields, the religious or spiritual dimensions of the lives of service users are not addressed, whether consciously or by default. It is, on this view, as if these professions have also undergone a sort of secularization in a way that renders them unable to address religion and spirituality in theory or in practice.

The second possible explanation of the apparent invisibility of religion and spirituality in the discourse of social work and human services is that in an increasingly multicultural world such phenomena can be regarded as potentially divisive. That is, the silence around these issues could be said to come not from an implicit acceptance that in a secular world such matters are simply private choices, but rather from an avoidance of the potential disagreements that would arise from open exchanges about such beliefs and values. As Midgley and Sanzenbach (1989) note, some forms of religious belief can be regarded as antithetical to professional ideas and values (compare with Azmi, 1997). These can be regarded as conservative or as fundamentalist, but however they are understood these approaches to religion usually tend to oppose the practices of social work and human services on religious grounds.

Alternatively, it may be that when practitioners hold quite different religious or spiritual beliefs to those of their service users it is more appropriate to ignore these in order to engage in practice on the basis of those ideas and values that are shared. This could be said to be not so much 'practical atheism' as 'practical agnosticism'. That is, it does not concern the exclusion of religion and spirituality as necessarily irrelevant but is more a way of suspending judgement about any understanding of these matters in order that public discourse can avoid tensions and disagreements that are both impossible to resolve and often regarded as not central to shared concerns around social well-being. Thus, whether or not these phenomena are significant for many individuals and communities, they tend not to be addressed explicitly.

Yet, at the same time, religion has played an active role in the development of the human service professions, in diverse ways. Both the traditions of casework, leading to counselling and other micro-level practices, and of community work, which from its earliest days was associated with policy development and structural change, have roots in the actions of the representatives of organized religions, such as clergy (Midgely & Sanzenbach, 1989, p. 274; Bowpitt, 1998; Payne, 2005, pp. 23–26). Moreover, just as the actions of religious groups and individuals within them have contributed to abuses and oppression, so too have they been part of more progressive developments, either in social well-being generally or in practices that came to form what are now professionalized as the human services. For example, as much as religious values underpinned European enslavement of colonized people, so too was this opposed and dismantled through the arguments of religious values (Anti-Slavery Society, 2008). More specifically, the actions of the Barnetts in London or Addams in Chicago in establishing Toynbee Hall and Hull House respectively, the forerunners of community work, are instances of religious values engaging with the critique of social structures and relationships and, at least in Addams' case, clearly working towards social justice (Reisch, 2004; Payne, 2005, pp. 37–38).

Whether the professionalization of social work and human services is regarded as 'taking over from' religion and spirituality or as building on and integrating religious and spiritual values, the construction of social work and human services is rationalist and scientific: in other words, it is modernist. Arising from this, there is another approach to religion and spirituality evident in social work and human services, which is the recognition of these phenomena as 'anthropological'. In other words, where they are recognized and addressed at all, religion and spirituality can often be regarded as facets of culture and/or psychological states. Therefore they are treated as 'facts' to be known about, especially when working with service users who are from a different cultural background to that of the practitioner. Thus they become part of a knowledge base, as informing cultural awareness and so contributing to 'cross-cultural competence' (see discussion of this notion in Chapter 5) (Graham & Shier, 2009, p. 230; compare with Dean, 2001; O'Hagan, 2001; Hodge & Limb, 2010). For this reason, Graham and Shier's observation (2009, p. 224) that much of the writing about religion and spirituality in relation to social work is produced in Western countries, and especially the USA, may be understandable. These are contexts in which the liberal politics of multiculturalism is much more dominant and this approach to questions of religion and spirituality can be seen as informing practice with 'ethnic minority' populations, in which knowing about service users' beliefs as an aspect or expression of culture is seen as valuable (Hodge & Limb, 2010).

Yet, if it is the case that many people, in modernist Western societies as well as other parts of the world, identify religion and spirituality as important phenomena in shaping their lives, to treat these simply as 'facts', or technical aspects of knowledge seems to miss out a whole dimension of human life (Canda & Furman, 1999; Furman *et al.*, 2004; Gray *et al.*, 2008). For example, there is the risk that this may lead to them being treated as superficial (in the sense of being on the surface) and so not addressed in practice. To understand how culture and values intersect and inform professional practice requires that religion and spirituality are recognized and addressed explicitly. The rest of this chapter seeks to look at how this can assist an understanding of the relationship between culture, values and ethics in social work and the human services. To do this, it focuses particularly on beliefs, ideas, practices and values, and addresses the specific institutions that commonly mark the domain of 'religion' only in so far as this adds to the analysis.

A comparative view of religion, culture and values

As has already been noted above, there is often a sense that social work and other human services professions derive from European or Western culture and so also can be regarded as having grown out of secularized Christianity. If the geography of these professional origins is accepted there is, however, a need to consider religious and spiritual roots more closely. Not only Christian but also Jewish ideas and beliefs have been part of professionalization in these fields, for example (Payne, 2005). Together with Islam, these religious communities are often identified in studies of religion as sharing a common set of beliefs and may be referred to collectively as 'the People of the Book' or as 'the Abrahamic faiths' (Berger, 2004; Dickson, 2004). The Jewish contribution to the development of social work and psychology, in particular, can be traced to the *diaspora* and Jewish presence in European and Western societies. While these religions clearly have many differences theologically, they share a common framework on an understanding of divine authority for the obligations that make up the moral dimension of the world (Hinman, 2008). In this sense, they point to a transcendent view of morality, in which community-sanctioned interpretation of tradition and teaching shapes ethical debate. That is, the source of moral authority lies outside any individual and has to be grasped through relationship with others in a recognizable community of belief. Nevertheless, these religions are marked by sharing a notion of the self as an autonomous entity, distinct even where it can only be fully known in relationship with other selves (Berger, 2004). It is this sense of self that runs through modernism and is often described as 'Western'; this is the view of self that can be immediately recognized in psychology, psychiatry, social work and other helping professions (again, whether or not this self can be understood separately from community). Moreover, the transcendental source of both morality and historical selves is also understood as a self, autonomous and in this sense 'personal' (Dickson, 2004).

Other religious or faith traditions take different approaches to such questions. From a comparative point of view, Hinduism, Buddhism and Jainism share a common underlying world-view. Moreover, just as Christianity and Islam can be seen as historical developments from roots in Judaism, so too can Buddhism and Jainism be seen as developments out of Hindu roots (as can Sikhism, although it took a different path on some key issues). Berger (2004, p. 22) distinguishes between these major groups of faith traditions in terms of their geographical origins, as the Jerusalem and Benares (or Banaras) religions, respectively, although he also acknowledges the important differences within these groupings. The key element of the 'Benares faiths' for a consideration of the ethics and values that underpin social work and human services is that they share a view of the self as transient, at least in so far as this relates to any particular manifestation in an historical person: in that sense the self is not 'real' and its autonomy is also transient. This view is grounded in an understanding of ultimate reality as 'not a self', so that the transcendental source of both morality and historical selves is impersonal and the idea of this source having autonomy simply does not make sense (Dhand, 2002; Dickson, 2004; Mohanty, 2007, pp. 64–65; Siderits, 2007, p. 293).

Any consideration of religion and spirituality needs also to look at those forms of belief and associated practices that are less easy to categorize. In many parts of the world such belief systems continue to be major sources of meaning for people and their communities, expressing deep truths and also conveying sets of ideas about what has come to be known as morality. These include African and Indigenous spiritualities, which to some extent share central features in an emphasis on community and relationship (often above and beyond individual selves) and in which human life is regarded as part of the natural world in a way that is distinct from either the Jerusalem or Benares faiths (Yellow Bird, 1999; Graham, 2002). Indeed, these spiritualities are not best understood as religions in that while they are socially organized this usually is not in the form of institutions that would be recognizable as comparable to the organization or practices of the other two focal perspectives (which, in this sense, have relative social similarities). As Graham (2002) notes with regard to African spirituality, it is indistinguishable from the relationships of community. For the Indigenous or First Nations peoples of (what is now) North America, the central concern of spirituality is identity with and care for and by the land on which a people live (Yellow Bird, 1999). In these terms, questions of self are not unimportant but the meaning of self cannot be separated from location in community, such as in the principle of *ubuntu* (Graham, 2002). From a Western perspective such a position can appear to be very similar to the 'denial' of the self in the Eastern traditions. Indigenous and African beliefs about the nature of ultimate reality also are difficult to translate into terms that make sense to the discourse of either Western or Eastern religion, although there are some apparent similarities. For example, in both African and Indigenous spiritualities there are narratives of the creation of the universe which then form the basis for morality and which connect people to each other and to ultimate reality through the relationship between land and people as part of that creation. From this, the parallels with the creation narratives in the Jerusalem faiths provides a potential basis for creating dialogue between African, Indigenous and other spiritualities (Rainbow Spirit Elders, 2007).

For social work and human services, these differences present some major issues. If religion and spirituality are regarded as a part of the life world of many service users, and also professionals, then this raises issues for the ways in which social work and human services are understood and practised. It may not be sufficient, for example, for the social worker, community worker or youth worker to 'compartmentalize' (Rorty, 1999, p. 270) this widely shared aspect of human culture from their concerns with the well-being of service users, their grasp of professional theory or, indeed, their understanding of themselves as practitioners. Yet in accepting that this is an aspect of being human that is relevant for human services, there remains the problem of how to engage more seriously with religion and spirituality while simultaneously accepting that these are matters on which everyone might reasonably hold divergent and even conflicting views. For this reason, addressing religion and spirituality explicitly raises ethical problems in the sense of asking how professionals can act well in relation to such differences and at the same time poses questions about ideas and values that can be found in the plural ethical stock on which professional ethics is built.

Religion, spirituality and practice

To examine further the questions that have been raised so far in this chapter, the following two hypothetical situations provide an illustration of the complexities involved. The first of these is located in a large regional town in an English-speaking Western country.

> Sylvia and Michael are two social workers employed in a government community-based children and families service. Michael has just returned to the office from a visit to the home of a family whose three sons (aged 14, 11 and 7) have been referred by their school and by the police. Not previously known to the police or to the social work agency, the boys have recently been caught damaging cars parked in the street. Michael, who is an atheist, is aware that Sylvia is a member of a Christian church, although this is not a topic of conversation in the office. One of Michael's concerns in the conversation that he has had with the boys and their mother is that she seems reluctant to accept professional help for the family because she wants to seek the intervention of the elder at the church that she and the boys attend. Michael's own view is that religion can offer nothing particularly useful for the lives of this family and he is concerned

that intervention by a religious leader will potentially make matters worse. Sylvia's response is that she cannot speak for all other faith communities, but she is aware that her own church employs some people who have qualifications in the helping professions. She wonders, therefore, whether it should simply be assumed that any intervention from a religious institution will be unhelpful or whether Michael's assessment is based on his own beliefs. Having agreed to differ on this point, Michael and Sylvia concur that there is a more serious problem in that if the boys continue this behaviour then such a choice for the mother will cease to be an option as she may be required by the police or a court to accept intervention. Michael wonders if perhaps Sylvia might be better placed to work with the case as she appears more comfortable in discussing religion. Sylvia's response is that any social worker ought to have the skills of working with service users whose belief systems are different to their own: 'think of it as cross-cultural practice', she suggests.

This interaction raises a number of questions. What happens when the beliefs and values of service users conflict with those of professionals who are providing assistance? Are there limits to how far it is reasonable to expect that professionals should engage with service users whose views they find challenging or even are ones that the professionals oppose? Is this simply a matter of working cross-culturally, as Sylvia suggests, or do such issues require a different understanding?

The second hypothetical situation is in India and concerns a meeting between Malathi, a health education worker, and Mansoor, who is a fieldworker with a social development non-government organization.

Malathi and Mansoor are meeting because they are working in the same part of a regional town, in which there are several areas where people live in considerable poverty. Part of the focus of the health education programme is to help families to become more aware of the risks faced by children. However, in these communities it is usual for children to contribute to family income through work that is dirty and sometimes dangerous, including scavenging for recyclable material on the streets and the local waste dump. The focus of Mansoor's project is to work with groups of families to assist them in developing small-scale income generation projects. Malathi has become concerned that one of the outcomes of Mansoor's project has been that children are being drawn into alternative labour, which, although not as high risk as working on the streets, can also involve health hazards. In any case, her agency's policy is also to facilitate children engaging with formal education at least at primary level. The community in which these projects are based has a substantial Hindu majority and a Muslim minority. Malathi, as a Hindu, and Mansoor, as a Muslim, agree that it would be helpful if the local religious leaders were to share the goals of their work. From their own religious upbringing, neither can see any reason why the local temple and mosque should not be invited to work together to support the projects, but Malathi and Mansoor are aware that in recent years there has been some tension between these faith communities, which partly came from differences of belief concerning employment opportunities, the types of work that people saw each other as appropriately engaged in and access to external support for such development. Neither Malathi or Mansoor agree with these exclusionary or sectarian views, but they agree that it may take time and effort to find ways to overcome this factor.

It must immediately be made clear that religious conflict as an issue faced by social workers and other human service professionals is not confined to these faiths or to this part of the world. As O'Hagan (2001), Maglajlic (2011) and Neocleous (2011), among others, have noted, there are many instances where religious belief and identity has played a part in conflict within and between communities in Europe in recent decades. The questions raised by Malathi and Monsoor's situation for practice are how such matters might impact on community-based interventions in a less extreme context, how religious ideas and the people who represent them might be considered as important in thinking about ways to engage in project work, and also, unspoken but implicitly there, the implications that this has for professionals who are members of particular faiths but whose roles require them to act with '[a] proper and positive sense of neutrality and clearly just behaviour' (Murphy, 2011, p. 162).

There are many threads and common dimensions in the questions raised between these two situations, even though one is in a Western context and the other in Asia. In many ways, Murphy's observation about 'positive neutrality' and 'just behaviour' sums up one of the central issues not only for considering religion and spirituality in social work and human services practice, but more generally for the 'self' of the practitioner in relation to values and ethics. That is, in working across all forms of 'cultural difference', including that which might be about religious and spiritual beliefs as Sylvia suggests above, there is a necessity to consider how the relationship between the professional role and the self is understood. In this sense, Sylvia is suggesting a response to this challenge that is similar to that being considered by Malathi and Mansoor, namely that working across or between belief systems requires the capacity to engage with difference.

This notion of 'cultural' difference applied to matters of religion and spirituality may be easier to understand in situations where there is a much longer history of multiculturalism defined around faith and belief, as is the case in a country such as India. By contrast, at least up to the twentieth century, Western countries have tended to be considered from within and without as monocultural in this respect. Although they have been the sites of religious conflict, this has mostly taken the form of 'sectarian' difference, which is not usually understood in terms of culture as such (compare with O'Hagan, 2001). However, in so far as the notion of 'cultural competence' can be considered plausible (see above), this might offer a way to begin to think about such questions if approached critically (compare Dean, 2001, with Hodge & Limb, 2010). Such an approach can be thought of as having three dimensions: how professionals relate to service users; how professionals relate to themselves; and how professionals understand the relationship between service users and themselves in social context.

First, the ethical principle of respecting persons can provide a foundation for being open to the world-views of service users, whether individuals, families or communities. This does not demand that a practitioner comes to agree with the service user, or even finds the service user's beliefs and values acceptable as such. What is required is openness to the service user's world-view; that is, being able to accept it at face value. Indeed, this does not necessitate 'knowing about' such world-views ('knowledge of another culture') but rather emphasizes the capacity to listen to the way in which service users express their own beliefs and values. Although this may sound like quite a traditional and orthodox concept, it runs counter to some ways of grasping 'otherness', especially in relation to matters such as religion and spirituality. Where these questions are considered as if they concern a form of anthropology, aspects of society 'to be known about', the result can be an imposition of such knowledge rather than listening to the person or group. It is not that knowledge does not provide some help, but rather that it is not sufficient to enable cross-cultural practice to occur. It is also the case that individual experience and world-views can differ widely within cultures. Hodge and Limb (2010, p. 271) give the example of assumptions that can be made about matters of spirituality among Indigenous North Americans, where the range of influences is such that there is often greater diversity and complexity than non-Indigenous professionals might appreciate.

Second, one of the major problems faced in social work and the human services for practitioners who are from a modernist, secular background (so, often, Western) is the lack of appreciation that culture is something that is an element of everyone's identity. Ironically, Hodge and Limb appear to make this sort of assumption in their ascription of 'culture' to those communities that are not part of 'the mainstream' (2010, pp. 265–266). In other words, we are all 'ethnic' but the language and experience of Western societies in particular is such that this word/concept is usually automatically attached to that of 'minority'. This can have a number of implications. It might lead to regarding culture or ethnicity as a deficit or a problem in itself. For the secular modernist, such as Michael in the above illustrative situation, this appears potentially to include religious and spiritual beliefs. Being able to consider oneself in this way can be a way of achieving integrity. For example, especially for practitioners from an 'ethnic majority' background, being able to reflect critically on the strengths of one's own culture, that is avoiding the arrogance or sense of superiority that can come from several centuries of colonialism or dominance, can provide a more confident basis for meeting service users and colleagues from other backgrounds in a respectful and open way. Without such respect, the pursuit of social justice can become illusive (compare with Maglajlic, 2011; Murphy, 2011).

Third, a critical but balanced understanding of oneself and one's own cultural background as something that is brought to the encounter with service users can then provide a basis for dealing with the problems that can arise from encountering oneself as 'other'. An example of the problems that can arise in this sense is that of moral defensiveness, sometimes referred to as 'white guilt', that can get in the way of ethnic majority practitioners working with those from ethnic minorities, or 'mainstream' workers with Indigenous service users and colleagues (Green & Baldry, 2008; Hodge

& Limb, 2010). So, such understanding might also include an awareness of the historical and current issues faced by a community, so that the context of individual and group experiences can be better grasped (Hodge & Limb, 2010, p. 271). Again, this is not simply about abstract knowledge but concerns the significance that such things have for individuals and across communities.

Considered from an ethical perspective, it would appear that issues of religion and spirituality present much the same challenges for theory and practice as do any other beliefs and values. Yet, as shown at the beginning of this chapter, this particular area of human life is regarded by some as having the potential to be socially divisive. It was also noted that the origins of social work and the human services can, at least partly, be explained in terms of the demise or silencing of religion and spirituality in the public arena through processes of secularization. So, making these matters the focus for explicit consideration requires that careful thought be given also to the ways in which this aspect of human life may be made more explicit in contemporary theory and practice in professionalized social welfare. It is to this question that the chapter now turns.

Ethical pluralism and a diverse religious world

In his discussion of ethical pluralism Hinman (2008) identifies three approaches to the relationship between religious and spiritual belief and reason in considerations of ethics. These are: the supremacy of religion; the supremacy of reason; compatibilism (religion and reason coexist). As Hinman goes on to explain, each of these broad positions contains variations in which different ways of looking at these questions are possible. While avoiding a definitive statement that one of these is the 'correct' view (Hinman's work is, after all, an argument for pluralism), the conclusion is that a plurality of positions is possible and that the capacity for people to hold divergent views in these things as well as on other moral matters is desirable. In this way, Hinman seeks to avoid both the universalist (there is one truth and this is it) and relativist (all truths are equally valuable) positions, although in this regard the former is the greater challenge to a pluralist approach (2008, p. 92). This challenge arises in a particular version of the 'supremacy of religion' position, where conviction about the truth of a belief leads to intolerance of those who think differently. Of course, holding to the truth of one's beliefs in itself is plausible – if beliefs are not true then why hold them? The problem arises from intolerance, that by holding to a truth it then becomes necessary to demand that everyone else also share this belief. Moreover, because such beliefs tend to be regarded as literal, it is difficult if not impossible to allow for others to hold different views. This position Hinman calls 'fundamentalism' (2008, p. 92), and he appears to apply it as much to the modernist implacable rejection of spirituality as to its religious variant. Rorty (1999, p. 157) makes a similar point when he says that '[s]cientific realism and religious fundamentalism are products of the same urge'. On this point Hinman and Rorty both regard the best of possible worlds to be one in which people are free to pursue the beliefs that make most sense to them and contribute to their well-being, up to the point where such belief starts to harm others. The problem, then, is how to find a way to live in such a way as to enable this to happen, when beliefs and values can make claims in the public space but do not necessarily coexist comfortably with each other. (This point is pursued in other ways in the following chapters.) Hinman's conclusion (2008, pp. 92–93) is to consider another strand of religious and spiritual belief, which he associates with an 'ecumenical' approach, one that is open to truths in other traditions and belief systems and which acknowledges its own limitations.

One aspect of the tension between a plurality of religious beliefs and the shared discourse of public life can be seen in the continuing contribution of religious organizations to human services, especially as this has been reformulated in Western countries in recent years as 'faith-based welfare' (Gilligan, 2010). The particular issue in this development has been the privatization of human services from state organizations to agencies run by particular religious bodies. While some criticism has come from those who are opposed to the way in which some faith-based organizations use volunteer workers rather than those who are formally trained, both for ideological and economic reasons, this move has also been attacked by secular or atheist groups because it is seen as introducing particular religious values to public social welfare (Gilligan, 2010, p. 69). Not only may faith-based organizations make some requirements about the beliefs of staff they employ but they are also perceived as potentially favouring particular approaches to social issues and problems. For this reason what is regarded by those within such organizations as the legitimate expression of their beliefs and values can be experienced by others as exclusionary and perhaps even as a form of the 'fundamentalism' to which Hinman and Rorty refer (see above). However, Gilligan (2010) also notes that the evidence for these concerns differs between the various commentaries and it also appears that in some cases interpretations may be at least partly related to the more general views about religion held by the commentators.

One such analysis is that of Nagel (2006) who points to the terms of the USA policies 'Charitable Choice' and 'Faith-Based Initiatives'. These contain regulations designed to ensure that: 'recipients must not be denied services for religious reasons nor may they be forced or urged to participate in religious action' and 'there has to be a comparable non-religious alternative, which recipients may chose in case they feel restricted in their (negative) religious freedom' (Nagel, 2006, p. 85). There are also balancing rights for services not to be discriminated against because of their religious base. However, Nagel also notes that in practice faith-based NGOs can be suspicious about external (secular, government) intervention into their procedures and external critics remain unconvinced about the extent to which the safeguards for service users actually operate (2006, p. 87). But he also argues from evidence in the USA that faith-based organizations actually tend to serve a different section of the population, as in the studies he summarizes as many as 75 per cent of service users in some agencies had not previously accessed services (p. 92). Other studies have likewise suggested that some faith-based organizations provide services to groups of people who are not otherwise catered for, especially those who might be thought of as 'hard to reach' (Cnaan & Newman, 2010). For example, another study found very few differences between faith-based and non-religious organizations in terms of organizational efficiency and other key factors that have driven this policy shift in the USA, but they did identify that faith-based organizations tended to address 'emergency needs' and to 'serve a more disadvantaged client population' (Reingold *et al.*, 2007, p. 274). The reasons for this appear to be complex and partly include the way in which some faith-based organizations provide services through funds they have raised themselves rather than solely relying on government grants and thus can have different criteria for rationing.

Another aspect of the work of faith-based organizations noted by Reingold and his colleagues is that for some, although by no means all, faith-based organizations the underlying purpose of engaging with welfare services is to encourage people to join their faith community (2007, p. 278). While restricting services to people within a particular community is prohibited by the relevant legislation where those services are publicly funded, the motivation of people who give their time voluntarily to work in such programmes cannot be ignored.

In contrast, however, Sercombe (2010) makes a very strong argument that irrespective of whether a service is funded by the state or a faith-based organization, it is inappropriate on ethical grounds for roles to be blurred (also see Green, 2010). In other words, any person accessing a service, whether it be receiving material assistance, personal help such as counselling, youth work or community development, should be able to understand clearly whether they are engaging with what could be described as a 'religious' activity or receiving a human service. As Sercombe puts it, 'not all work with young people done from a faith perspective is youth work' (2010, p. 32). In other words, in considering whether a service is actually a religious provision as opposed to a human service it is important to examine the focus. So, if the aim is to encourage people to belong to a faith community, or to assist them in their spirituality, then it should be seen clearly as a religious activity. This does not mean ignoring questions raised by service users about such matters, or of masking the fact that a service is run by a faith-based organization, for example. What it does require is to focus on the service user by addressing their definitions of their needs and problems.

There is a very clear connection here between Sercombe's position and Koehn's understanding of professional ethics that was discussed in Chapter 3. To recap, for Koehn (1994) the virtuous professional is the practitioner for whom the centre of their focus is the service user, as distinct from the professional's own interest in knowledge and skills for their own sake, for example, or the status, income or other benefit that can derive from professional work. For practitioners who have a religious motivation to undertake such work this means setting aside their own belief systems, as much as it might involve health professionals making the patient their primary focus as opposed to the perfection of a particular clinical technique or the discovery of new knowledge about a condition (good as these things may be for other reasons).

From this understanding, the illustrative situations described earlier in this chapter show aspects of the problems that may have to be resolved in practice. For Sylvia and Michael, considering the needs of a family where a single mother wishes to seek help from a religious elder to respond to challenging behaviour exhibited by her three sons, the question of the mother's values and wishes is not something that can be ignored if practitioners are to act well. It seems appropriate, on this view, for Sylvia to question Michael's dismissal of the mother's wish to consult the elder as a possible form of personal bias and to try to concentrate instead on whether the person involved actually has the capacity to help the family. As Burton and Bosek argue (2000, pp. 102–104) if practitioners are to work with a service user's value structure as a starting point then brushing aside religion and spirituality simply as evidence of immaturity or psychological disturbance is at best an inadequate response and at worst is ethically poor practice. To use their terms, when this happens it is not just religion and spirituality that become ethical issues but also professional beliefs and knowledge. Burton and Bosek give an example of the family of a cardiac patient sacrificing a chicken at the hospital bedside in a healing ceremony (2000, p. 101). The initial response of clinical staff was to ask for the family to be removed from the hospital. However, when this event was explored further a means was found to enable the family to perform their own ceremonies as they saw fit while maintaining the clinical integrity of the hospital setting, by conducting a more limited version in a specially cleared space that could be sterilized afterwards. As their discussion emphasizes, this did not require anyone to accept claims that they found unacceptable but rather to find ways of respecting each other and working together for a shared goal, the well-being of the patient. As Burton and Bosek note (2000, p. 105), this is a problem that was resolved; while this may not always happen they argue that ethics that attends to religion and spirituality whether as a source of values or just as a social fact needs to have such accommodation as a goal. For Michael this perspective would mean seeking to find a way of working with the religious elder, irrespective of his continued personal difference of beliefs.

For the situation faced by Malathi and Mansoor the ethical challenge is somewhat different. Here the differences between religions appear to be the ethical challenge. However, in concrete terms the practice implications are very similar. That is, as Malathi and Mansoor have agreed, the social development goals for the neighbourhood will be achieved more effectively if the two different religious communities are able to work together. Thus, whatever the religious or spiritual beliefs or affiliations of the practitioners, focusing on ways of enabling members of the two different groups to meet and share their concerns and their efforts to achieve these goals is appropriate. This might even require consciously, if carefully, arguing against claims that either community cannot have such connections with the other. Again, the point is not to challenge core beliefs by engaging in religious debate as such (and here too arguments for agnosticism or atheism must also count as beliefs concerning religion) but to find sufficient shared commitment to common action in a context where religion and spirituality form central foundations for the values of those who live in the neighbourhood.

It will be clear from this discussion that what is being proposed is a version of the pluralist approach that Hinman (2008) calls 'compatibilism' (see above). This not only means that neither religion nor rationality are regarded as the only plausible set of values, but that different religions also can be accepted as reasonably having a place in a diverse society. This must also be acknowledged as a distinct ethical position. It is open to critique and dispute as much as any other. However, this is the position on religion and spirituality that most effectively contributes to the achievement of the wider direction of the argument in other parts of this book, namely that in diverse societies, whether these are understood as local, national or international, a primary goal of social work and the other human services professions must be to promote dialogue and ways to find the sharing of values to the extent that this enables people to live well alongside each other. In this sense the approach is not only pluralist but also pragmatic (compare Hinman, 2008, with Rorty, 1999).

The final word on this matter can be given to Versfeld (2005) who uses the metaphor of a shared meal to describe such a goal. This image is most apt, in that shared meals play a central part in many religions, as well as in families and communities, and some of the problems of different traditions and positions in finding ways to accommodate to differences of belief and values can be expressed clearly in considering how a meal might be shared without anyone being required to subordinate to other faith communities or belief systems those values that they hold as most important. As Versfeld (2005, p. 183) observes:

> The ecumenical [that is, inter-religious] problem is how to eat with others, how to borrow ingredients and techniques from others and how to be ethnic without being exclusive.

8 Ethical pluralism and the democratic urge

Social work and human services and democratic values

In the previous chapter the implication of religion and spirituality for thinking about professional ethics and values was examined. In particular, the discussion looked at the way in which diverse beliefs and positions may create challenges for social work and human services practice and considered some ways of thinking about whether the accommodation of differences is possible. This chapter pursues the question of differences further, broadening the discussion to examine ways in which the relationship between wider social and political structures and the ethics and values of these professions is impacted by cultural diversity. It considers the relationship of social work and human services to particular political values and explores ways in which the idea of multiculturalism can inform thinking about culture, values and ethics in this field. Arguments for anti-racist practice and also for culturally specific services have become increasingly important for social work and human services, and these ideas are also discussed in depth. This discussion also draws on the notion of anti-oppressive practice.

Early forms of social work in particular, but also the antecedents of other types of human services, can be said to have embodied the values of liberal democracy quite explicitly. The writings and practices of Jane Addams (2002 [1907]) in the USA are a particularly clear example of this. Addams argued that only through the pursuit of democracy would social work be able to address the issues and problems with which it is concerned. This quite clearly included advocacy for change and development in policy and social practices at the widest level, which requires engagement with social structures and governmentality, alongside interventions with individuals and groups. Legislation and policy to control child labour was one of Addams' key examples (2002 [1907], p. 76). Another was her continual efforts to promote peace (Payne, 2005, p. 40, records Addams as the only social worker to have won a Nobel Prize, for peace campaigning). Addams' view of democracy was that of a society in which individuals and groups are free to exchange ideas, to question, criticize and seek change and so to play a role in political and social structures. However, for her this was above all an *ethical* claim, one that was legitimated by being grounded in the pursuit of social equality, emphasizing that as all human beings are moral equals so this should be reflected in social relationships, whether of education, employment, the family or public life. For Addams, these are all areas of ethical concern for social work.

In Europe, also, early social work was very much part of the emerging modern forms of liberal democracy. In the UK the foundation of professional training for social workers was influenced by the arguments of social democrats and socialists such as the Fabian Society as well as by more conservative perspectives such as the Charity Organisation Society (Payne, 2005). Payne also notes the relationship between the beginnings of professional social work and social and political reform focused on social welfare in other parts of Europe, notably Germany, Belgium and the Scandinavian countries. He argues that the German approaches even influenced social welfare developments in Japan (Payne, 2005, pp. 44–45). However, his discussion of these countries emphasizes the more conservative dimensions of these trends, especially the role of social welfare in mitigating social unrest.

Clearly, therefore, social work and human services have to be understood in relation to social and political values. The history of these professions in the twentieth century and the way in which they have developed around the world (Healy, 2008; Hugman, 2010) suggest that there may be particular connections between them and certain types of social and political structures. The question that is raised is whether social work and human services can best develop (or, indeed, only develop) in liberal democratic societies. From this there is then a further question about the implications of any such connections for practice and policy in culturally diverse societies. For example, in Chapters 4 and 5, the core values claimed by the key international social work and human services organizations (IFSW, IASSW, ICSW) were identified as social justice and human rights. As discussed there, these values, in particular human rights, have been challenged from various positions, in both the global South and North, as inappropriate. One example of this is the assertion that such values are 'Western' and therefore irrelevant to cultures such as those of Asia. Although this argument has been strongly rebutted by Kofi Annan when he was General Secretary of the United Nations (Annan, 1997), it continues to be raised in other contexts, as noted in Chapter 5. The implications of this debate, however, is that it raises the question of whether professionalized social work and human services can only be developed within particular social and political structures, notably those that may be understood as forms of liberal democracy.

The idea of liberal democracy encapsulates key social and political values that have been identified previously. In summary, these are based on the moral autonomy of the individual, leading to the notion that legitimate government has to have the consent of those people who are governed. These are ideas that developed at the start of the European Enlightenment, for example in the work of Hobbes and Locke, and find their significance as ethics in Kant (MacIntyre, 1998; Hinman, 2008). Thus, the claim that the idea of human rights is associated with liberalism has some historical basis. So, given the importance of human rights as one of the core values claimed by social work and human services, the relevance of this relationship is that it raises the question of whether such professional practices and institutions fit with diverse social and political values. In other words, are social work and human services inescapably 'Western' because they are liberal in this sense? This question will be addressed first by exploring the analyses of two theorists of cultural diversity whose work has so far had relatively little impact in thinking about social work and human services, Kymlicka (1989, 1995, 1997) and Benhabib (2002, 2004, 2006), and then asking how their conclusions can assist in understanding debates that have been introduced in previous chapters.

Kymlicka: culture and citizenship

The context of Kymlicka's analysis is that of Canada. The population of Canada is ethnically diverse, including the First Nations peoples as well as those who are either themselves migrants or are descended from migrants from many different parts of the world. The socially and politically dominant cultures are those from Northern Europe, most particularly the UK and France. Kymlicka's central concern, therefore, is how to reconcile questions of citizenship in such a liberal democracy, which includes a wide variation of ideas about social and political values (Kymlicka, 1989). Most importantly, it must be accepted that the claims of ethnic minority groups to a particular standing with regard to the right to be different from the dominant culture, including values about such things as family life and relationships, religion, dress and so on, may even at times conflict with those of the dominant culture. However, underlying this situation is the plausibility of collective rights for minority cultures (Kymlicka, 1989, p. 145). For Kymlicka, individual autonomy is not an end in itself but a means to the end of pursuing those projects and practices that are valued for their own sake (1989, p. 12). It is at this point that liberalism and pluralism come very close together. Moreover, these projects and practices are grounded in the cultures of those people who value them. So, where community or cultural membership is claimed as a core value then this should be accorded the status of a right, because it is this which gives meaning to the things that people pursue. In other words, for some people the opportunity to live as a member of a cultural community is one of the most important things in their lives. This can be seen in projects such as the formation of culturally based community organizations or in practices that include food, dress and religion, with associated rights and social recognition. This, in summary, is the basis of multiculturalism.

   Such a position immediately raises further questions. From the position of liberalism the central problem arises when a community claims the right to values that are separate from the mainstream but at the same time asserts that members of the community are not to be able to exercise the same degree of freedom (Kymlicka, 1995, pp. 152–153). The rights of cultural minorities in liberal democracies cannot extend to the internal restriction of community members' rights to question dominant values, to favour different values or, indeed, to leave a community. Nor do minority rights stretch to one community oppressing another through denial of their rights to cultural integrity. In this sense, Kymlicka's argument can be said to advance the idea that in liberal democracies the collective rights of ethnic groups parallel those of individuals, in that as the rights of any member of the society are bounded by the rights of others so too are the collective rights of ethnic groups. This argument leads to a plural perspective, because it enables each person to pursue those things that they find to be of value in themselves and so supports a wide plurality of goods; in turn this enables a plurality of cultural values to be sought. This plurality includes the ways in which both individuals and communities address the values and rights of others and thus this position is advancing a 'diversity of approaches to diversity' (1995, p. 190).

Kymlicka (1997, p. 64) is also very clear that cultural pluralism does not support ethnic separatism. For him, it is the lack of multicultural policies and practices that actually promotes and sustains marginalization and claims for separateness, because without the possibility of a plurality of values and the recognition of difference in ethnicity minority communities may feel encouraged to cut themselves off from the majority ('the mainstream'). The implications of this view for ethno-specific human services are explored in detail below. One possible exception that Kymlicka (1989, pp. 145 ff.) considers is that of First Nations, Indigenous or Aboriginal peoples, whether in settler societies such as Canada, the Americas, Australia or New Zealand or in other parts of the world where such a status is not so widely recognized. (For example, there are ethnic minority communities in various parts of Asia and Africa who may be regarded as Indigenous in this sense, but where the ethnic majority community has been established for very long periods of time.) In order to redress historical inequalities and to balance up the advantage that non-Indigenous people have in being able to make life choices and to pursue their own cultural values, special civil and political rights are required by Indigenous people. This position, Kymlicka argues (1989, p. 192), is a working through of Rawls' (1972) theory of justice in that it creates fairness between different communities in terms of the social and political conditions that they enjoy in order to pursue valued projects and practices.

Benhabib: cosmopolitanism and particularism

Writing in a somewhat different context, that of the UK, Benhabib approaches similar questions to those of Kymlicka but from another perspective. Where Kymlicka starts from a consideration of political arguments for liberal multiculturalism, Benhabib is concerned to 'mediate moral universalism with ethnic particularism' and 'legal and political norms with moral ones' (2006, pp. 19–20). In other words, she wishes to find a balance between shared values and the differing value claims of diverse cultural groups, in which difference thrives out of a common base, and at the same time to make clear the links between civil and political values and ethics.

Nevertheless, Benhabib's starting point is quite close to Kymlicka's notion of the limits on the rights claims of cultural communities, in that she considers the purpose of multiculturalism to be the promotion of justice and freedom and not the preservation of cultures as such (Benhabib, 2002, p. 8). This is because culture matters to people as the basis on which they can live their lives and understand their own identities. Benhabib (2002) takes issue with Kymlicka in that she considers his view of cultural communities may lead to a sense in which ethnic identities can become treated as monolithic. In contrast, she asserts that 'there are competing collective narratives and significations that range across and form the dialogue of cultures' (2002, p. 60). That is, all cultures can be seen as containing internally plural perspectives and as changing over time; thus in examining the relationship between cultures within shared societies it is important to recognize that they are dynamic. This can make intercultural dialogue as complex as it is necessary.

Benhabib (2002, p. 101) is also very clear that the analysis of culture and values cannot ignore the way in which social relations are gendered.

> There is little doubt that women's concerns and the status of the private sphere expose the vulnerability of multicultural arrangements and reveal the unjust moral and political compromises, achieved at the expense of women and children, upon which they rest.

The same argument can be applied to other distinctions, such as those of sexuality, age or disability. Yet this does not mean that ethnic communities should be polarized between the preservation of cultural traditions and the promotion of the autonomy of individuals. Instead, in multicultural societies, which are necessarily pluralist, wider social institutions can respond by recognizing and supporting the diversity within particular ethnic communities. In the end, Benhabib's argument connects again with Kymlicka's in that she advocates that multicultural pluralism, both between and within ethnic communities, must rest on egalitarian reciprocity, voluntary self-ascription and the freedom of association and of exit (2002, pp. 131–132).

From this point Benhabib (2004, 2006) goes on to argue for a 'cosmopolitan' view of the moral relationships between cultural communities. This is the same foundation as that which informs Sen's (1983) and Nussbaum's (2000) concepts that are discussed in Chapter 4. Put simply, this is the view that primary values, both political and ethical, can be seen to be shared around the world and, following Kant, to provide the basis for seeing members of all communities as part of a common humanity (Benhabib, 2006, p. 20). Thus the question in not whether human rights and social justice are culturally specific but, rather, what meaning people claim for them within their own cultural context. As with Kymlicka, Benhabib argues that it is not legitimate for the leaders of ethnic communities to claim the right to distinct identity and values only to then use this right to deny the rights of those who are members of their community or of other communities. This applies both to membership of distinct cultural communities within a given nation state and also to cultural relationships between nations. However, perhaps paradoxically, the same communities which make claims to cosmopolitan values 'are also based on the cultural, historical, and legal memories, traditions, and institutions of a particular people and peoples' (Benhabib, 2006, p. 169). In other words, although the autonomy of ethnic communities relies on strong liberal democracies, the identity of each community is founded on its traditions and customs and this creates political and ethical questions of acceptance and accommodation for liberal democracies as it does for each cultural community. Thus there is a continuing tension between particularist traditional values and the universalist liberalism that provides the social space in which such values can be pursued.

Multiculturalism and anti-racism

Relatively little attention has been paid in social work and the human services to the ideas of Kymlicka and Benhabib, at least in English language writings about these professional areas. Indeed, there is not much explicit discussion of multiculturalism as a concept in these fields. Rather, the notions of anti-discrimination, anti-racism and anti-oppressive practice are much more well developed, at least in English language writings (Thompson, 1993; Banks, 2004; Dominelli, 2008, 2010; Clifford & Burke, 2009; Sercombe, 2010; Soydan, 2010). There are very close connections between these ideas and practices, but these are not always either obvious or straightforward. Nevertheless, it will assist the present consideration of values and ethics in these professions to ask some questions, in particular about how the two notions of multiculturalism and anti-racism intersect.

Dominelli (2008, pp. 8–9) defines racism as a social construction of bias, in which some social groups discriminate and oppress others on the basis of perceived physical differences, notably skin colour, the shape of facial features and so on. She makes the important point that in terms of biological science all human beings are one 'race', that of *Homo sapiens* (p. 8). But racism is more than a simple representation of difference: it is grounded in drawing political and social implications from such ascriptions, in which dominant groups legitimize their subordination of others on the basis of perceived difference. In reality, racism is not simply about physical characteristics, but conflates these with culture and then applies its conclusions in exclusionary and dominating social relationships, action and structures.

This leads Dominelli (2008, pp. 12–16) to identify three forms of racism, which interact with each other in social relationships: individual racism; cultural racism; institutional racism. The first of these is what many people understand as racism, in the negative attitudes and prejudices held by individual people about those who they perceive to be inferior because they are different. Second, cultural racism is the set of ideas that make up a shared world-view, usually embedded in language, religion, philosophy, family relationships and so on, which assign relative worth between cultures. An example of this is the belief in colonial Europe that Europeans were superior to all other 'races' on the basis of a view of their own culture as being superior. Such views continue to be held, and may be held by people from other cultures as well; where they constitute racism (as opposed to personal prejudice) is in situations where such ideas can be used to oppress others. Institutional racism is where the political and social structures of a society routinize oppressions and discriminations based on 'racial' differences in the institutional arrangements of public life. For social work and the human services, there are many such areas, including education, health, housing, employment and income support, personal social services and community development. Professional organizations and practices are also part of this aspect.

Some of the hypothetical practice examples provided in previous chapters display clear elements of racism. For example, in Chapter 1 the situation of a young woman in a youth service who wears the *hijab* (head scarf) is presented, whose response to taunts from other young people is to ask for ethnic-specific sessions. This example was used to raise questions in that chapter but was left without resolution. How individual workers and how the service as a whole respond will reflect their understanding of and responsiveness to the racism in this situation; it will also provide an indication of the extent to which multiculturalism is being realized in everyday life. Similarly, in Chapter 2 differences in expectations about child-rearing practices were presented, with a child being referred to a child welfare agency because of bruising produced by physical discipline. The resolution of this situation, that a social worker is allocated to both provide advice and also to supervise the situation, is experienced by the family as potentially having a racist rationale. The extent to which individual, cultural and institutional racism can be identified in each is partly a matter of perspective, although some degree of individual racism is quite clear in the first example.

In both cases the solutions available to the practitioners can appear to be relatively straightforward. For example, the youth centre workers can engage the other young people in developing awareness around the rights that each person has to dress in ways that are appropriate to their culture. In the meantime, they can support the young woman in question and challenge racist statements as inappropriate and unacceptable in the youth centre. With the family, it may be possible to engage in dialogue around cultural norms of child-rearing in ways that do not simply dismiss the family's sense of their own culture and yet also help them to grasp the expectations of the wider community (Robinson, 2007). As previously noted, the child protection legislation in this country cannot be set aside on grounds of culture, even if it must be applied through culturally informed and sensitive practices.

Yet, at the same time, both these ways of proceeding contain quite specific claims to a particular way of responding. The first response makes a claim that cultural differences of dress are not simply 'acceptable' but are to be regarded as a 'right'; the second starts with the assumption that physically hurting children to discipline them is 'wrong'. So these two different sets of assumptions together raise the question of whether every challenge to someone on the basis of something that they may regard as part of their 'racial' or cultural identity, by a person or institution that is seen as dominant, is always best understood as racism. In these examples, challenging a young woman's wish to wear ethnically specific forms of dress can be regarded unambiguously as racism, while challenging certain child-rearing practices might or might not. This basic difference can be explained in terms of the positive and negative implications of acts: in the first instance the young woman's claim to ethnic identity is harmed if she is denied the right to wear appropriate head covering; in the second instance the child's interests are seen as being harmed by physical chastisement. In addition, the former can also be said to have one primary subject, the young woman, as there is no one else whose interests are directly affected. In contrast, in the second instance the interests of both the child and the parents are directly affected, and it is the latter who feel a moral hurt through their perception of cultural racism. France is currently the only country in which the right to certain forms of culturally specific dress is the subject of restrictive legislation (full-face head covering, such as *niqab* and *burka*, are banned by law from being worn in public places), while critics argue the choice of such garments should remain a matter of individual freedom (BBC, 2011). However, legislation concerning limits to parents rights to use physical chastisement now exist in many countries and take no account of claims to cultural norms. Such examples show the limits to multiculturalism in liberal democracies, in that it is at these points that variations in the resolution of value conflicts are found.

Thus, these examples point to the question 'what are the conditions in which the exercise of power by social work and human service professionals, for example, should be understood in terms of racism and those in which it should not?' It is here that the central paradox of both liberalism and pluralism is encountered, namely that although diversity is valued and difference is not simply tolerated but positively embraced, there is a limit. Not everything goes. The idea of multiculturalism implies social structures that enable different ethnic communities to pursue their own valued projects and practices in conditions of equality, what Modood (2007) calls 'positive difference'. Yet in areas such as child welfare, services for young people and other community services, many of the goals of practice are strongly contested because these are important areas of life in which the dominant, mainstream values are often asserted through law, policy and practice. Consequently, for some service users and communities any practices and policies that are not based on their own views of the world will be regarded as oppressive and thus racist, while for others this may not be an issue. Indeed, both Modood (2007) and Dominelli (2008) note that differentiation, prejudice and discrimination may not be equally expressed or experienced between various ethnic minority communities. It may even be said that there are different racisms. The question that follows from this is whether in a society that is comprised of many cultural communities the way of resolving the question of potential racisms in social work and human services is to create ethnic-specific practices and policies, so that each person and group may consider that they are being served in a culturally relevant way. It is to this question that the chapter now turns.

Cultural diversity and ethnic-specific services?

At this point in the discussion it will be useful to return briefly to the arguments of Azmi (1997) that were noted in Chapter 5. This comes from an analysis of the traditional Muslim community in Toronto, Canada. Azmi's argument is that the use of modern liberal concepts in such a traditional community is a form of ideological 'missionary activity' (p. 116). According to both Kymlicka (1989, 1997) and Benhabib (2002, 2006), such a claim can only succeed in so far as those aspects of the traditional culture are freely entered into by the people involved and do not make any claims on other cultural groups or the overall society that would undermine their right to have their values supported. Understood in this way there are limits to the extent to which ethnic particularism can be achieved for all those things with which social work and human services are concerned. The application of laws in relation to the possible harm of children is one such a case.

It is in this context that arguments for ethnic-specific social welfare services have to be considered. These may take the form of institutionally separate provision, whether in entirely distinct services or programmes, or they may be found in making common services or programmes available in ways that are tailored to the particular needs and interests of different cultural communities. In some post-colonial 'settler societies', such as Australia, Canada, New Zealand and the USA, there may be some separate legislation relating to First Nations (Indigenous or Aboriginal) peoples, as advocated by Kymlicka (1989) (Weaver, 2004; Blackstock & Trocmé, 2005; Munford & Walsh-Tapiata, 2006; Green & Baldry, 2008).

There are many examples of ethnic-specific services or programmes, including those concerned with children and families (Evans & Garwick, 2002; Blackstock & Trocmé, 2005), mental health (Lau & Zane, 2000; Griner & Smith, 2005; Akutsu *et al.*, 2007), disabilities (Evans & Garwick, 2002), care of older people (Hikoyeda & Wallace, 2002; Radermacher *et al.*, 2009), and community development (Baines, 2008) (also see Thyer *et al.*, 2010). Certain common themes can be seen in these discussions, which can be taken as the parameters or 'boundaries' of how cultural communities are addressed in practice and policy:

- the meaning of 'ethnic-specific' can be regarded in very broad terms, such as 'Asian', 'Latino' or 'Muslim', or very specifically by country of origin, such as 'Afghan', 'Greek', 'Sudanese', 'Vietnamese' and so on;
- ethnic-specific services may be provided as extensions of 'mainstream' services or as alternatives;
- questions of ethnicity sometimes refer to all aspects of culture and sometimes stand in place of 'minority language' issues;
- there are closely related but distinct issues raised for social workers and human service professionals in these services who are themselves members of the relevant cultural communities.

The range of possible variations within these parameters makes analysis of ethnic-specific services quite complex. For example, Radermacher *et al.* (2009, p. 58) note that both specific services that are extensions of mainstream provision and separate services may exist alongside each other, for the same types of human services needs and in the same neighbourhoods. However, in terms of values and ethics there are some clear inferences that can be drawn.

First, there is widespread agreement that ethnic-specific services are regarded by service users as beneficial. Problems may be understood more easily, solutions and interventions are more easily tailored to cultural expectations, issues of sensitivity to barriers in using services (such as 'shame' experienced in using mental health services) may be more easily managed, and direct experiences of racism (whether overt or perceived) are reduced (Lau & Zane, 2000; Evans & Garwick, 2002; Blackstock & Trocmé, 2005; Akutsu *et al.*, 2007; Baines, 2008; Radermacher *et al.*, 2009). In this way ethnic-specific services can be regarded as providing members of cultural minority communities with greater access to social work and human services than might otherwise be possible. Given that these studies echo findings elsewhere that members of such minority communities disproportionately regard mainstream services as inaccessible, irrelevant or hostile (see, for example, Dominelli, 2008), such services provide a way of remedying disadvantage. In this respect Kymlicka's argument (above) about the way in which culturally separate structures may be to the advantage of minority communities, in that the disadvantages that they face in the overall society are moderated if not fully ameliorated, can be seen to be relevant. The ethical argument is one of social justice as a balance, in which it is acceptable that those who are worst off should receive apparently disproportionate attention, because the goal of equality defined as 'everyone can access the same services' may have (unintended) consequences of creating an actual inequality when those services are actually inappropriate to culturally specific needs.

Second, it is also clear that all the programmes and institutions that these studies examine recognize and allow for the choices made by members of minority ethnic communities, in that no-one is denied access to the mainstream services if they choose to seek them. Some human services professionals may seek out members of these communities, and encourage them to consider the culturally specific provision, yet this is not to create a forced segregation but rather because they are aware that many members of these communities do not access services at all even though they have relevant needs (Akutsu *et al.*, 2007; Baines, 2008). In this way choices of 'membership' and 'exit', in both a practical and a moral sense, are respected.

Third, however, some studies also caution that in times of reduced social welfare spending, services that are seen as 'special' can be the disproportionate subject of financial and other constraints (Blackstock & Trocmé, 2005; Baines, 2008; Radermacher *et al.*, 2009). This may apply particularly to those services that are separate as opposed to extensions of mainstream provision. One of the reasons for this, identified by Baines (2008, p. 126) is that at times of a general reduction in the levels of public provision of social welfare the arguments for ethnic-specific services are more fiercely contested. Such an issue demonstrates how the concept of social justice is not always either understood or accepted. In Rawls' (1972) formulation of criteria for justice in conditions of inequality, he argued that inequalities may be just if they can be shown to be to the benefit of the least advantaged. On these grounds, separate services could clearly be said to be fair and reasonable, and it is this principle to which Kymlicka is referring when he argues for such an approach for Aboriginal peoples. The argument of these studies, and the services that they describe, goes further than this because they also advocate for cultural communities who are not Indigenous; thus the moral and political claims of these services are more highly contested. To be fair to Kymlicka, his concern is to limit the legitimacy of more radical claims for separateness, of the kind advocated by Azmi (1997), which might imply entirely separate 'societies within a society'. The one exception Kymlicka allows is that of Aboriginal peoples because of the claims they have in relation to the territory on which the society now stands. They have been 'dispossessed' in a way that cannot be said for any other group. Ethnic-specific human services provision is not such a claim, but a more limited way of responding to the needs of communities who are already often marginalized and whose members may lack access to the same levels of provision as others in the society.

It is also possible that objections to ethnic-specific human services represent forms of racism, whether intended or otherwise. As Dominelli notes, the maintenance of cultural values and distinctiveness can be seen by critics as in some way failing to be part of the wider society and so of losing legitimacy (2008, p. 169). Liberal democracy in this sense can be seen as embodying the claim that 'we are all in this together', emphasizing commonality and unity. Nevertheless, as Dominelli also notes (p. 46), such distinctions should not be imposed on people but should relate to their own perceptions of their lives. The example that she gives is of children with mixed-race parentage who tend in a country such as the UK (and in many other Western countries) to be regarded as 'black', whereas their cultural identity and belonging may embrace the backgrounds of both parents. This is not to suggest, as Dominelli makes clear, that the reality in Western countries for people who are not recognized as 'white' can be understood without reference to the concept of 'black' as a political issue (compare, for example, with Robinson, 1995). However, although this is a socially structured understanding, it is part not only of social relationships but also of the psychological experience of members of 'black' minority communities (Robinson, 1995) – and, it may be added, as a corollary, as part of the social and psychological experience of 'white' members of the cultural majority in that 'black' cultural identities and values may come to be regarded not only as 'other' but also as 'inadequate' in some way.

This observation points to a very particular debate in relation to culture, ethnicity and 'race' – that of the family and especially of children within families as they are regarded by social work and the human services, in practice and in policy. It is to this aspect of the debate that this chapter now turns.

The family, children and culture

In Chapter 4 Nussbaum's (2000) arguments concerning the factors that are necessary for a flourishing human life were reviewed. To recap, these are the capability of achieving: life of normal length; bodily health; bodily integrity; senses, imagination and thought; emotions; practical reason; affiliation; relationship to other species; play; and control over one's environment. While Nussbaum's concept emphasizes the shared nature of these capabilities among all humanity, it also requires recognition of the way that these appear differently in each culture. (The discussion returns to this point in Chapter 9.) One of the most important aspects of human life in which these capabilities are exercised is that of having and rearing children, with life-long implications for intergenerational relationships (as discussed in Chapter 2 concerning 'filial piety', that is moral obligations to older generations, especially blood-relatives). Indeed, there is evidence that the idea of 'family' can be regarded as one of the few firmly established 'anthropological absolutes', although it is crucial to emphasize again that what family looks like in different cultures varies considerably (compare Nussbaum, 2000, with Baxter, 2005). The right 'to found a family' is enshrined in Article 16 of the *Universal Declaration of Human Rights* (UN, 1948), which goes on to say that '[t]he family is the natural and fundamental group unit of society and is entitled to protection by society and the State'. Measures by the state that permit or require agencies to intervene in this group or unit, therefore, must have strong and widely supported reasoning to be seen as just and reasonable.

Robinson (2007) argues that practitioners should become more familiar with the differences of values between the cultures with whom they work. However, this does not mean that all social workers and human services professionals have to aspire to encyclopedic knowledge about all cultures. Dominelli (2008, p. 82) suggests that what is required is the capacity to listen carefully to any service user's account of how they understand their own culture and to work with the diversity of values in which the practitioner's own values are experienced by service users as 'other'. In this sense, competence in working cross-culturally is best understood as an aspect of reflexive practice, as opposed to simply a technical skill. Heterogeneity *within* as well as between cultures has to be recognized, although this can make it harder for practitioners to be confident that they are not going to misunderstand claims to culture as the basis for interactions with service users. One such aspect is that of the way in which socio-economic class differences have cultural dimensions, as discussed in Chapter 5. But even taking this into consideration, it is still reasonable that families that share such objective characteristics may, even so, have different approaches to the same cultural or ethnic background, with implications for child-rearing and other parts of family life. Thus the capacity of the practitioner to be reflexive is the most helpful way of looking at a positive understanding of professionalism in cross-cultural practice.

The challenge of cultural diversity for social work and human services practice with families and children also has to be seen in the context of law and policy. In so far as these do not provide the basis for differential responses based on minority community membership, then the question for practice is that of how to work within legal and policy requirements to provide effective and appropriate responses to diverse service users. As Pierce and Bozalek (2009) note from a cross-national study involving South Africa and the USA, the definition of child maltreatment and neglect, as well as legislation and policy, differs between these two countries. In South Africa in the post-apartheid era (since 1994) child maltreatment has been increasingly recognized as an issue in and for all ethnic communities, whereas in the USA this has been the case for much longer. Perhaps as a consequence of this, as well as other policy and practice differences (such as reporting systems), the largest number of known instances in South Africa concern sexual abuse, while in the USA neglect is the largest category, with physical assault being second in both countries (Pierce & Bozalek, 2009,

p. 120). This also appears to be affected by particular experiences of poverty, dislocation, the history of communal and political violence in South Africa and so on (Barbarin, 2003; Lalor, 2004). A major difference between advanced industrial countries and those that are 'developing' or 'in transition' is whether child labour or children begging is regarded as abuse (Pierce & Bozalek, 2004).

Pierce and Bozalek (2004, p. 818) note that how different factors are perceived as child maltreatment is affected by '(1) cultural differences in childrearing practices and beliefs, (2) idiosyncratic departure from one's cultural continuum of acceptable behavior, and (3) societal harm to children'. Nevertheless, such studies demonstrate that in both Africa and North America, and across different cultural communities in both places, the broader question of the safety of children and their right not to be violated is regarded as important. All cultures have strong values about the care of children and while many details may differ, at their most basic these values support the health and development of children (see discussion in Chapter 2). Using Nussbaum's approach to human capabilities, it may be argued that maltreatment destroys a child's expectations of achieving key aspects of living a valued human life, such as bodily health and integrity, emotions, practical reason, affiliation, play and control over one's environment. These are part of the factors identified by cross-cultural and cross-national studies such as those of Pierce and Bozalek (2004, 2009), Lalor (2004) and others. From this it can be seen that there are some strong bases from which to have cross-cultural dialogue about children's rights and needs in relation to those of families and other social actors (Clifford & Burke, 2009).

One particular situation in the UK in 1984 highlights many of the difficulties faced in micro-level practice in this field, that of the death of Jasmine Beckford (Blom-Cooper, 1985). This was the situation of a girl of Caribbean ethnic background who was in the care of the state but placed with her family as part of a reintegrative case plan. Jasmine died as the result of injuries inflicted by her father. In the subsequent inquiry it emerged that the social workers employed by the government agency with statutory responsibility for Jasmine's well-being had chosen not to insist on seeing her after her father had refused to allow them to do so in a routine visit to the family's home. Their argument was that in doing so they were respecting Mr Beckford's self-determination and, as the family were 'black' and they were 'white', this represented anti-racist practice. The inquiry concluded that this was not acceptable (and, indeed, went further and took this description of social work ethics at face value, proceeding curiously to criticize social work as a profession) (Blom-Cooper, 1985). In terms of the analysis presented in this present discussion, the conclusion that this was not good practice is correct, as it does not accurately grasp either professional ethics or anti-racism. What was missing was a more nuanced understanding of the cultural claims being made (such physical harm of a child by a parent is no more morally normative in the Caribbean than it is in European cultures) and how the statutory role in relation of the rights of the child could have been enacted in an anti-racist manner. (It also represents a serious misunderstanding of professional ethics and principles such as self-determination.)

It is this latter point in particular that connects professional values and ethics in social work and human services with the question of how multiculturalism can be achieved in a democratic society. As noted above, it is not only members of cultural minority communities who may be critical of professional interventions and try to resist them, as socio-economic class can play a comparable role as a factor in how people regard receiving statutory child welfare practice. Safeguards on such practices, therefore, have to take into account not only the question of ethnicity but also of other factors, including socio-economic class, gender, disability, sexuality and belief, to ensure that the rights of parents are maintained as much as possible to the degree which is consistent with the rights of children being protected.

Multiculturalism and democracy: the challenge for social work and human services

To return to the question with which this chapter began, it is the case that in so far as the professionalization of social work and the human services has origins in the development of modern democratic societies, with implications for equality between people of different class backgrounds, men and women, and irrespective of belief, ability, sexuality or age, that they will be seen as embodying particular cultural values. It is also part of the history of social work, in particular through the twentieth century, that as it became adopted more widely around the world this process has often failed to address cultural and social differences in practices and in policies (Midgley, 1981; Gray, 2005; Hugman, 2010). The spread of these ideas and practices has often accompanied shifts towards more democratic social relationships and structures, although to differing degrees. The critique of inappropriate approaches to policy and practice tends usually to at least stop short of a defence of totalitarian governments, for example. Indeed, it usually concerns arguments for more diverse practices, such as community work and social development, instead of a more uniform application of individualistic social welfare administration. While an individual-level focus is obviously congruent with liberal democracy, the more macro-level practices also tend to promote democratic values.

For these reasons, social work and the human services cannot be regarded as politically or culturally neutral. In the terms of theorists such as Kymlicka and Benhabib (see above) these professions are part of the wider society in which cultural minorities can plausibly maintain their right to recognition by also accepting the limits to these formed by the rights of others, as also occurs for individuals within liberal democracies. The argument for ethnic-specific services is just and reasonable in so far as it fits within this framework, which would include the possibility of members of cultural minority communities accessing 'mainstream' services should they wish to do so. The argument for practices (and supporting theory) that are relevant to a member of any particular cultural community, in contrast (and paradoxically to some critics), is a universal claim in that it embodies core professional values and ethics, such as those of respect for persons, human rights and social justice, and so is also just and reasonable even if on a somewhat different basis. To achieve this may mean that differences in practice are not only developed but also are actually affirmed as good.

This chapter and the previous chapter have developed further the arguments that were set out in Chapter 6, which are those of value pluralism. As argued there, the position of pluralism suggests that goals of 'tolerance' and 'acceptance' are central to social work and human services embracing diversity. Yet, as has also been noted at several points, there are some limits to tolerance and acceptance, reached when these professions assert some values as primary. So to examine the implications of this in more depth, the next chapter explores the way in which pluralism and diversity may present a paradox for professional values and ethics.

9 The paradox of value difference and ethical pluralism

Value difference and ethical challenge

Earlier chapters have examined universal and relative ideas about values and ethics and then considered a pluralist response. Then, in Chapters 7 and 8 the implications of these ideas for social work and human services in thinking about religion and spirituality and about multicultural societies have been explored. In this chapter the discussion returns to the question of pluralism as an approach to values and ethics, with a specific focus on the implications for social work and human services practices and policies. Of particular concern here is how social work and human services may respond to the challenges of cultural diversity for shared professional values and ethics. After looking at questions of formal professional codes of ethics, with particular attention to the recognition of Indigenous and ethnic minority cultural values, the discussion returns to issues of power and authority that have been raised in earlier chapters. From this a pluralist approach to ethics is proposed as the effective way of engaging with cross-cultural practice.

A central difficulty presented by the idea of pluralism is that it requires social workers and other human services professionals to be able to work effectively and positively with different value perspectives while at the same time holding a clear position as members of the respective professions. Most especially: how do members of these professions respond to others whose value positions are different; and how do members of these professions who hold differing values achieve a shared position within the profession? This in turn raises the question of whether pluralism is a matter of 'tolerance' or of a deeper 'acceptance', in which diversity is not only taken as a fact and 'worked around' but is embraced in order to become part of the values of these professions. From this concern, it can also be seen that the issue of diversity and difference has implications for how the forms of social work and human services can be compared between countries and cultures, taking further the arguments of Chapters 4, 5 and 6.

To recap on the central issue of cultural diversity for social work and human services, the claims made by professions to overarching statements of values and ethics imply a universal understanding of the goals and purposes of these practices (see discussion in Chapter 3). Examples include the national codes of ethics for social work, youth work, community development, community health professions and so on (such as: BASW, 2002; YACWA, 2003; ANZASW, 2008; NASW, 2008; AASW,

2010; compare with: Fry & Johnstone, 2002; Banks, 2006; Sercombe, 2010) and also the international 'codes' and statements (such as: IFSW/IASSW, 2004; ICN, 2006; IUPS, 2008). Within these documents there are some attempts to address the differences of cultural values between communities within each society as well as between members of the professions. However, only a few appear to make substantial, concrete attempts to incorporate such differences in formal ethical statements. Most notably, the national codes for social work in Aotearoa-New Zealand (ANZASW, 2008) and in Australia (AASW, 2010) include explicit recognition of the value and ethical implications of Indigenous peoples both as service users and as members of the professions.

The ANZASW *Code of Ethics* (2008) is distinctive, in that it is written in two languages (Maori and English) and seeks to embody the implications of the Treaty of Waitangi (te Tiriti o Waitangi) (section 3). This treaty is the founding document of the modern nation of Aotearoa-New Zealand, signed in 1840 by Maori chiefs and representatives of the British Government. To embrace the implications of this historical background, the ANZASW code commits social workers to understand the bi-cultural history of the country, to seek appropriate ways of working with members of all communities, to develop social work beyond monocultural theories, practices and institutions, and to seek actively to be anti-racist in their practice (ANZASW, 2008, section 3.1). At the same time, this code also makes explicit reference to the IFSW/IASSW (2004) *Statement of Ethics* as a foundation, as well as having an entire section on the principle of human rights (ANZASW, sections 4 and 5).

The Australian code (AASW, 2010) was extensively reviewed in order to address both developments and ethics within the profession and an increased responsiveness to the position of Aboriginal Australians, both within the profession and as service users. The code begins with a 'preamble' that acknowledges the status of Aboriginal and Torres Strait Islander people as the First Australians (p. 5). Subsequently, specific statements are made in relation to relevant aspects of ethics, for example in a section detailing 'general ethical responsibilities', where it states that:

> Social workers will value the unique cultural knowledge and skills, different knowledge systems, history, lived experience and community relationships of Aboriginal and Torres Strait Islander peoples, and take these into account in the making of decisions.
>
> (section 5.1.1.c)

Similarly, under the following section on 'culturally competent, safe and sensitive practice' the code specifies:

> Where possible, social workers will seek guidance regarding service development and delivery from community members, mentors, advisors and recognized Elders from culturally and linguistically diverse communities, Aboriginal and Torres Strait Islander communities and other cultures and communities.
>
> (section 5.1.2 (i))

In addition, the ethical responsibility to 'recognise and challenge racism [...] through the use of anti-racist and anti-oppressive practice principles' is stated (section 5.1.2 (l)). In forming this code, the voice of Aboriginal and Torres Strait Islander social workers was represented by a separate national working group as well as through membership of the review committee (personal communication). In this way the AASW sought to model the principles that are described in the code.

In contrast, the social work codes of Canada (CASW/ACTS, 2005) and the USA (NASW, 2008) give priority to the large cultural minorities of these countries by publishing French and Spanish language editions respectively. So, while both countries are settler societies facing similar issues of the relationship between Indigenous peoples and social work and human services, they appear to be responding to questions of culture in a different way to the approaches of Aotearoa-New Zealand or Australia. For example, in the USA the code states that social workers 'should understand culture and [recognize] the strengths that exist in all cultures' (NASW, 2008, section 1.05 (a)), and have knowledge of the cultures of their clients and demonstrate the capacity to work cross-culturally (section 1.05 (b)). In common with the Aotearoa-New Zealand and Australian codes, the Canadian and USA codes contain explicit requirements about social workers being aware of social diversity and related questions of social justice and being able to practice appropriately in a multicultural society (CASW/ACTS, 2005; ANZASW, 2008; NASW, 2008, section 1.05 (c); AASW, 2010). This points to the way in which such aspects of practice concern values, not simply techniques. They are both goals and the methods of reaching them, ends as well as means.

This is not to say that all matters of the recognition and appropriate response to such issues are regarded in any of these countries as having been resolved. As has been noted at many points in previous chapters, statements of ethics may be aspirational as much or even more than they are descriptions of fact. Both in Aotearoa-New Zealand and in Australia there continues to be criticism of the reality of the lives of many Indigenous people (Briskman, 2007; Green & Baldry, 2008). Similarly, in Canada and the USA the French and Spanish speaking minority communities regard recognition as yet to be fully achieved. It should also be noted that there are Indigenous members of these professions in Canada and the USA for whom the lack of distinct recognition remains a major problem (Yellow Bird, 1999; Blackstock, 2004; Weaver, 2004; Blackstock & Trocmé, 2005; Yellow Bird & Gray, 2008). While this is not only a matter of ethical statements, the lack of recognition in these central professional documents can be taken by some as an indication that wider practice and policy implications are not recognized.

From a pluralistic perspective it may be reasonable that there are differences of approach between Australasia and North America, as although these regions share much in their histories, they also have separate paths of development. For example, Nussbaum observes that the strong legal prohibition in Germany on denial of the Holocaust of the mid-twentieth century makes good moral sense, while a similar limitation in the USA would confront the particular national understanding of the value of free speech (Nussbaum, 2002, p. 133). From this argument, it may be

concluded that debates about the primacy of Indigenous peoples as cultural minorities in professional ethics and practice must be resolved primarily at the national
level, as in each country the nuances of history and current social institutions means
that different responses may be appropriate. Nevertheless, the claim of Indigenous
people in settler societies appears to be very strong, even where there are other
minorities who also make plausible claims to distinct recognition, including recognition of the claims of women on grounds of gendered oppression (compare with
Nussbaum, 2002, p. 126).

All of these developments in thinking about formal ethical statements represent
forms of separate (or 'special') treatment of cultural minorities in order to redress
disadvantage and to promote social justice. In rethinking professional ethics in
these ways social workers are seeking to promote social justice, which is claimed as
a primary value for the profession, and in so doing these statements come to
embody the arguments of theorists such as Kymlicka (1989, 1995; see Chapter 8)
that separate treatment is justified in these circumstances, even though it appears to
favour one group or community over others. This is the idea that in order to redress
any disadvantage it may be necessary to provide something that is different, separate or 'more' than is provided for other social groups, thus creating an apparent
'inequality'. However, what seems to be an inequality is just or fair precisely
because without it the disadvantage cannot be redressed. In this sense, by engaging
in these ways with the situation of Indigenous peoples or of other cultural minorities these professional bodies are enacting their own statements of value and so
achieving integrity.

Such an approach is often considered as deontological, because the arguments for
it have been grounded in the ideas of Kant, for example, by Rawls (1972) and by
Kymlicka (1989, 1995, 1997). Yet there is a strong similarity between the notion that
justice is best protected by attending to the rights of the most disadvantaged groups
in a society and the arguments from utilitarianism, such as those of Singer (2002).
That is, a utilitarian approach would also support this conclusion by seeing the overall benefit to the society as greater than if one group or community continues to
experience extreme disadvantage. Indeed, as Hinman (2008, p. 255) points out, there
are many instances in which arguments based on duty to principle and those based
on consequences reach the same conclusions in terms of the right actions that should
follow. Therefore making such comparisons can also be understood as a way in which
agreement about what is good can be achieved. This makes such arguments very
strong. From this it can be concluded that the instance of special attention to the
situation of Indigenous peoples in professional ethics is very clearly a good development for many reasons.

Yet attention to such matters in formal statements is only part of the way in which
social work and human services can address the ethical challenge of value differences,
important as such statements may be for making goals public. In practice there can
be a challenge arising from value differences that has also to be addressed: how members of these professions can attend to differences of values between themselves,
between themselves and service users, and between different communities, while

adhering to the idea of shared professional values. It is to this question that this chapter now turns.

Difference, choice, authority and power

Social work and human services around the world share very similar functions. Although a precise definition of a profession such as social work seems at times to be elusive (compare with IFSW/IASSW, 2000/2001), in broad terms these professions have developed in order to assist people in resolving problems of social life. Yet there is a crucial distinction to be made between those problems that are defined as such by the people (individuals, groups, communities) who can be said to be experiencing them, and those that are defined in relation to these people by others. What this means is that the perception that there is a problem may be that of people with whom the practitioner will work, or it may be that of another entity such as the practitioner her- or himself, another professional, a government agency or other social institution and so on. Some people become service users because they seek services, while others are either brought to the attention of social work and human services or even compelled to receive an intervention whether or not they agree that there is a problem that concerns them.

A basic way of understanding this distinction is to use the notions of 'voluntary' and 'involuntary' service users. Certainly, these concepts are useful in terms of the power of the state through law to compel a person to 'receive assistance'. So, from this point of view it might be reasonable to say that whether or not the person's cultural background means that such a service is normative is irrelevant. It is not their choice to be a service user. On these grounds, such a question is meaningful only for the voluntary service user, who can make choices about whether or not to seek help and, if so, where to look for it. However, although this perspective does begin with a reasonable assumption (there is a difference in whether an intervention is chosen by service users or is mandated by authority) it oversimplifies the way in which factors such as authority, choice, freedom and so on are actually experienced and the impact of this on people's responses to professional services. There are three elements to this question, which need to be considered in turn.

First, even when the intervention is statutorily mandated, it still has to be relevant and (hopefully) effective. For example, simply because a young person is mandated by a court to participate in a youth offenders programme, and so to 'receive' counselling, psychology, social work or youth work, this does not take away the individuality of that young person and their capacity to engage with the intervention in their own way. How the young person understands what is said and done, indeed how they approach their engagement with services, will be grounded in their culture. So although it may be appropriate at the social or political level to argue that the treatment of young people who are found to have broken the law should not depend on their cultural background, how professionals respond to the person must do so. Attending to how each person understands their culture is part of engaging with them in a helping role. This is an example of attending to 'the person in their social context', in which 'individualization' of interventions does not mean blaming disadvantaged people for their disadvantage but ensuring that the particularity of a person's circumstances are appropriately recognized and taken into account.

Second, simply using this sort of distinction does not resolve whether the statutory basis of intervention is appropriate to a multicultural context. In other words, it is important for an ethical response for professionals to understand the legal, policy and organizational framework within which they are working. At its most confronting, this concerns whether or not the practitioner regards the laws, policies and procedures that shape their practice as culturally biased or racist. It may not be these things themselves that are racist, but their implementation. Many studies have shown that in multicultural societies the members of ethnic minority communities are often the subject of greater attention in the enforcement of laws and controlling policies and procedures (compare with Dominelli, 2008, pp. 91–96, p. 138, pp. 142–146). While it may not always be possible for individual practitioners to challenge laws and policies in their entirety, in this instance, in relation to cultural equity, it is the responsibility of professionals to be involved in such debates and to seek appropriate changes, so they can add their experience to a collective voice. Individuals may also make career choices based on their views about these things, for example working in advocacy and campaigning roles, or in policy and research work, as opposed to more direct work with individuals and families. Most importantly, social work and other human services professions can advocate for and support mechanisms through which the voice of groups, such as Indigenous peoples and other cultural minorities, can be heard in the processes of policy and law formation. This is the realization of the ethical codes discussed above (compare with AASW, 2010, section 5.1.2 (i)).

Third, this two-fold (or binary) distinction of 'voluntary/involuntary' misses the relevance of the power of professions, agencies and so on over those who are experiencing problems in social life (Hugman, 1991; Clifford & Burke, 2009, pp. 71–76). While it is at least possible in principle for someone who is a voluntary service user to decline what is offered, the social relationships of needing to ask for help may make this less easy than it appears. The service user is in a vulnerable position in relation to professionals and agencies, because it is the latter who control access to what is needed to deal with the problem. This may be expertise, knowledge or resources, or a combination of these; it will often include the capacity to make and implement decisions. Moreover, most users of social work and human services are in the lower socio-economic sectors of society, so that they are likely to be multiply disadvantaged in relation to those from whom they seek help (compare with the discussion in Chapter 5). This places additional ethical responsibilities on professionals, to seek to use their power to enable people to find appropriate solutions to problems rather than obstructing them (Clifford & Burke, 2009, p. 73). Attention to cultural relevance is a central aspect of the use of professional power. The arguments about the cultural appropriateness of 'non-directiveness' may be an example of this. The dominant perspective among Western-trained social workers may be to seek to be non-directive as much as possible, but this can be experienced as unhelpful if the service user feels impeded by a professional who will not give clear advice (compare with Nimmagadda & Cowger, 1999; Robinson, 2007, p. 172).

Whether service provision can be considered voluntary or involuntary on the part of the service user does not remove the question of cultural difference for professionals in social work and human services. The challenge, therefore, is to be able to work with an understanding both of the shared values of a profession, and the legal and policy framework of practice, while also attending to the service user, including their cultural background and the values it contains.

The cultural particularity of professional values?

Another major challenge of cultural difference for professional values and ethics is in the apparent notion that culture can, or indeed should, be treated as a monolithic and unchanging phenomenon. To address this point the discussion will first consider differences within as well as between cultures, and then proceed to examine the implications of cultural change for values and ethics in social work and human services.

Claims about what it is to 'be' a member of an ethnic group tend to emphasize those aspects of a culture that are held in common (Jenks, 1993). So what it is to 'be Australian' or 'be American' can be described, as may 'being Chinese' or 'being Arab', or again 'being Muslim'. Yet immediately a problem of conceptual clarity is encountered, in that the first two examples relate specifically to nation states, the next two to what might be regarded as ethnicities that can exist cross-nationally, while the final example is primarily an identity based on religion. Moreover, within each group there are major differences, between those who have a view of their culture that seeks to preserve traditions and those who moderate their understanding according to new social, political and economic circumstances. There may also be sub-groups, so that differences arise between socio-economic class groupings, or regionally between various parts of a country. In the case of Chinese or Arab identity, this may be influenced by which country a person was born and resides in, and similarly for Muslim identity. Indeed, it may be found that people construct multiple identities, in which they may refer to being Australian, Arab and Muslim, giving priority to various aspects according to their relevance in context (family relationships, work, the local community, religious practice and so on) (compare with Modood, 2007). Assumptions that a cultural identity is fixed and that it must contain certain characteristics is usually termed 'essentialism' which, as Modood notes (1997, pp. 91–93) is an inaccurate way of understanding culture because it is unhistorical and sociologically inadequate. Such a monolithic way of understanding the world is termed 'reification', in that it treats an interpretation of experience as a fixed, concrete reality.

It is for this reason, for example, that arguments against 'cultural competence' in social work and human services, such as Dean (2001) must be seen not as a rejection of the need to attend to culture as the basis of values, but as a rejection of 'reification'. This refers to ways of thinking that ascribe to something that is an idea or an understanding the property of being a concrete fact having clear boundaries and being indisputable. Dean (2001, p. 623) gives the example of herself as a 'white Jewish'

American woman working with a family from a minority community, in which the process was a not a matter of locating the 'correct' meaning of their culture and simply applying this knowledge – what Dean calls 'American "know-how"' (p. 624). Rather, it was that of learning about the ways in which family members, most especially the children who were the focus of her involvement, viewed their own culture and their experience of the wider society. In doing so, Dean saw herself as an active participant in the process, also bringing her own culture to the relationship, so that through this interaction both the family and she were able to change their understanding and from that to try to seek ways of achieving change.

Cultures in dynamic change

A further problem with the 'reified' or 'essentialist' view of culture is that it does not recognize historical change. Such an approach takes culture as something that is static. It assumes that 'this is how the culture is', with no awareness that it is most unlikely always to have been the same and may be subject to further change. The counter view, that culture is dynamic, can be considered by looking at some of the ideas that underpin social work and human services as professional activities.

One such example is that of responses to domestic and family violence. As has been noted in previous chapters, arguments have been made that professional interventions in such situations in cultural minority communities constitute invasive intrusions of the mainstream culture into those minority groups (Azmi, 1997; also see Yip, 2004). At the same time, the laws and policies that mandate such interventions represent the outcome of hard won arguments within the wider society. The public acknowledgement of domestic and family violence as a social issue that requires such intervention is relatively recent in the mainstream cultures of Western countries and in many ways can be seen as something for which legitimacy is not necessarily accepted by all sections of the mainstream culture (Hugman, 2008). As was discussed in Chapter 5, this may often have socio-economic/class dimensions, with a sense of arguments against 'interference' in families being couched in terms of the defence of working class families against the power of the state. However, first, it should not be assumed that domestic and family violence is an issue confined to the more economically disadvantaged sections of society (for example, see: Peter, 2009). Second, the public recognition and acceptance of this issue as a social problem that requires intervention is relatively recent. It is possible to date it from the work of the first 'women's refuges', such as the one in London in the 1970s established specifically for women seeking to leave violent partners (Pizzey, 1974).

As Hugman (2008) argues, such mainstream interventions and services were regarded by critics at the time as 'undermining the family'. This type of problem can be regarded even still as 'regrettable, but it's just how things are' – in other words, claims continue to be made in some parts of the mainstream society that such a phenomenon is normative. Yet there is also a strong thread of Western culture that argues against this, instead asserting that a good life includes being free from the fear of personal attack and injury, especially in one's home and from one's closest relatives.

This view has both religious and secular aspects, but can equally be claimed as authentic Western culture (Hugman, 2008).

The point here is that cultures change. Similar developments might also be observed in relation to child abuse, the abuse of adults who depend on others for personal care and so on (Roberts, 2000; Gallagher, 2004; Doe *et al.*, 2009). Indeed, social work and the human services have a long association with social and political action to create many such changes. It is less than 200 years since it was regarded as culturally normative in Western societies for some people to own other human beings as slaves, or to force children to undertake dangerous and degrading work. It should be noted that early forms of professional social work and human services, such as the Charity Organisation Societies and the Settlement Houses, were allied with social movements that included political reformers and even artists and writers such as, in the UK, Charles Dickens, much of whose work can be regarded as containing a thread of critical commentary on social injustice.

Modern social work and human services continue to contribute to the pressure for such developments, both in Western countries and elsewhere in the world. Slavery continues in many parts of the world (see, for example: Anti-Slavery Society, 2008), and social work and human services professionals are involved in various ways in working to end it. For example, these professions are among those who are employed by agencies involved in working with national governments to change law and policy concerning human trafficking, and with community groups in campaigning against this; they are also involved in providing assistance, such as counselling and services to assist with settlement of people who have been trafficked (Cox & Pawar, 2006; Healy, 2008; Hugman, 2010). The same can be said about the involvement of social work and human services in working against the use of children in dangerous and degrading work, as well as the abuse and neglect of children in other types of situation. Each of these phenomena can be said to be normative because they are 'traditional' and attempts to change them are resisted in local contexts. Yet at the same time, simply to criticize professional practices that oppose such phenomena as 'neo-colonial' ignores the extent to which people who are also part of the local culture may well be part of the movement for change and welcome the introduction of professional skills and knowledge in achieving such change. It should not be assumed that all professional social work and human services practitioners in such work are from other cultures; but even when they are, they may be welcomed *by those who stand to gain from change*. Opposition to development and humanitarian aid can be understood in the same way.

This is the point of the debate: opposition to cultural change has to be considered very carefully. It may be a reasonable defence against external interference, or it may itself be an attempt to hold on to advantage gained at the expense of the disadvantage of others. This is the significance of Annan's (1997) comment about the tendency of the principle of human rights being resisted as Western imperialism being a reflection of national or local exploitative vested interests. Within this debate, it must be remembered that in so far as the professionalization of social work and human services is considered a product of Western societies, they developed out of cultural change in their own original settings and were actually part of that change – as they continue to be. While it is the case that many forms of practice that have been shared with other parts of the world may be culturally inappropriate or insensitive (Midgely, 1981; Gray & Fook, 2004; Hugman, 2010), this does not invalidate the way in which practices that are appropriately modelled by, with and for people in their own situations may plausibly play a role in cultural change.

So, in the situations described by Azmi (1997) or by Yip (2004) among others, it may well be that social work and human services are regarded as incursions by cultural forces representing another, dominant culture and, moreover, one from which many expressions of hostility to the minority culture have been experienced. The pluralist argument is that this is reasonable if at the same time it is also possible for all cultural positions to be open to reconsideration and debate and if individuals are free to reject the claims of tradition, especially in matters of personal safety and well-being (compare with Benhabib, 2002, 2004). In the terms set out by both Kymlicka (1989, 1997) and Benhabib (2002, 2004) minority identity or status could not, in this way, exempt groups from the requirements of law and policy that needs to apply to everyone in order to secure the basis of such safety and well-being (for example, child protection legislation). At the same time, there is a moral and political responsibility on the part of state agents, such as the human service organizations that have the operational mandate in an area such as child protection, to seek to act in ways that sustain the integrity of minority cultures as far as this is possible while still fulfilling the statutory function, through anti-oppressive practices.

The paradox of pluralist values and ethics

Responding appropriately to the integrity of cultural groups while also recognizing that traditions are neither monolithic nor static reveals the potential paradox that lies at the core of a pluralist approach to values and ethics. A version of this paradox was outlined in the previous chapter, in noting that a cultural community cannot claim the right to difference of values and then deny the same right to its individual members without undermining its own claim. The problem here is how such a community may exist within a wider society and receive the benefits of that society while also being separate on matters of core values. There is a direct parallel here with Hamilton's observations about the value of freedom, which poses the question of how a person can simultaneously be an individual and part of a group (Hamilton, 2008, p. 314). One solution is that the community or the individual freely accepts limitations on their freedom. This, Hamilton is suggesting, is what most people do in modern, economically developed societies. The alternative is to seek a genuinely separate existence, which in reality can only be attempted by an entire country, such as in recent times by Cambodia, and currently by North Korea and Myanmar (Burma). Each of these societies has only succeeded in separating from the international community to the extent that it almost completely denies equivalent freedom to individuals, often to the point of genocide or other atrocities.

There are practical implications of such attempts to run societies against the prevailing values of the international community, such as in the work that ensues in responding to refugees. However, for most social work and human service practices, the implications of pluralism in this 'freedom paradox' are to be found in questions about the extent to which cultural differences should be 'tolerated' or 'accepted'. In a clear descriptive account of pluralism, Hinman (2008, p. 55) argues that pluralism of cultural values cannot lead to the relativistic position of 'anything goes': there have to be some limits beyond which even the committed pluralist will not go. As Hinman puts it, '[i]t is also important, at least in cases of egregious moral wrongdoing, to speak out against offenses wherever they may occur, whether in one's own or another culture' (ibid.). His instances are those areas that are immediately identifiable to social work and human services as central to their concerns, namely 'children, women or [other] minorities (whether these are racial, ethnic or religious minorities)' (ibid.). By egregious, Hinman means those values or acts that can be considered outrageous by agreement between a variety of robust ethical approaches as unacceptable. So, for example, domestic and family violence, or the abuse of children can be agreed in this way as outrageous, because such acts deny the person's humanity, fail to produce utility, demonstrate vices rather than virtues, are contrary to the teachings of most religions and so on.

Where the same test produces agreement that values or acts may be judged to affirm humanity, produce utility, demonstrate virtues and so on, even when they may be unusual or strange, then they should be embraced as representations of diversity. Hinman (2008, p. 55) suggest that 'tolerance' is the minimum aim, where this is seen as each culture giving others sufficient room to pursue their own values. However, 'tolerance' might also imply merely 'putting up with' and beyond this, where possible, positive acceptance is the mark of a more genuinely diverse society. To be sure, 'putting up with' is preferable to inappropriate hostility simply on grounds of another position being unusual or strange, but pluralism encourages the effort to go further and to give value to difference as part of what it is to be human. This does not imply that cultures have to accept each other's values, but to be able to appreciate as good that each culture has sufficient social space to pursue its values. Positive acceptance or affirmation of diversity implies a recognition that all positions gain from the unique features of each contributing to the total of human experience.

The implications of these two positions for social work and human services are quite clear to the pluralist. In relation to the former, practitioners should feel confident that their task is to protect and to promote the interests of those who are vulnerable, albeit while still seeking to respect cultural diversity as much as possible. In the latter, when invited to intervene practitioners should seek to develop ways of working, through means that are culturally sensitive and which affirm difference (Robinson, 2007; Dominelli, 2008; Clifford & Burke, 2009). 'When invited' here should not be challenging, as in any voluntary service provision the 'social mandate' of social work and human services is the consent of service users (compare with Hugman, 2005). Without such consent professionals lack the authority to act (although, as noted above the giving of consent is not of itself without certain problems).

It is in relation to phenomena that lie in between these two positions that problems still remain. For ethical pluralists, this may be because the ways in which different perspectives approach questions of value can be too far apart for agreement to be reachable. Under such circumstances, the values or practices of some communities may be considered unacceptable to others and where agreement is not possible then whether these then become regarded as 'outrageous' must be subject to public debate. What is of central importance here is the differing capacities of professionals and service agencies on the one hand and service users on the other, especially those of cultural minority background, to define the boundaries between 'different' and 'wrong' (compare with Healy, 2007). Unless these boundaries are open to review and discussion from many points of view there is a risk that minority perspectives become silenced.

How is this to be achieved? Again, Hinman's model of ethical pluralism provides a possibility. There are, he argues, two other principles in addition to those of tolerance or acceptance and of opposing that which is widely agreed as grossly unacceptable. These are fallibility and understanding (Hinman, 2008, pp. 54–56). By fallibility he means that although it is often necessary to make judgements between cultures about what may or may not be acceptable, this should be done 'in a spirit of humility and self-reflection' (ibid.). Cross-cultural dialogue should be exactly that, as this implies communication *between* people. In this sense the principle of fallibility does not require someone to be lukewarm about their own values, but to avoid dogmatism that prevents listening to other perspectives. For example, it is entirely possible that what have long been considered core social work and human services values are inadequate for responding to cultural difference and that it is these professional values that need to be rethought, rather than it being assumed that other values are deficient. Instances of this can be seen in the arguments about the understanding of non-Western families in Western countries and appropriate practice responses, whether these are in Indigenous or migrant communities (Blackstock & Trocmé, 2005; Robinson, 2007; Dominelli, 2008; Green & Baldry, 2008; Clifford & Burke, 2009). Being open to such arguments and seeking appropriate changes does not mean that social work and human services abandon concerns for those who are vulnerable. Rather, it requires that all such values and practices are open to questioning (which is also congruent with the position argued above in relation to the claims of communities in relation to individual members). For members of dominant cultural communities it is sometimes difficult to remember that everyone brings a cultural position to such an encounter (in other words, everyone has a culture); but this can only make the need to be conscious in addressing this point more urgent, it does not remove it.

This leads to the principle of understanding (Hinman, 2008, p. 55). This principle requires that in order to make cross-cultural judgements it is necessary to look very carefully at the values and practices of other cultures, beginning with the perspectives of members of the cultural community themselves, including internal community variations and differences. For Hinman, unless this happens dialogue will not be successful. What is meant here by 'understanding' goes beyond scientific and professional knowledge, important though that may be. There are many instances of such knowledge being inadequate precisely because cultural assumptions have not been recognized (for example, Robinson, 2007, pp. 24–30). This idea connects with the traditions of social work and human services in seeking not only to know about service users' lives in the abstract, but to gain insight into their lived experience.

These principles can assist social work and human services in thinking not only about values and ethics in local practices, but also in the international sphere. This can be seen not only when practitioners work in locations other than their home country, such as in development or humanitarian work (Healy, 2008), but also in the relationships between social workers and human services professionals in different parts of the world (Hugman, 2010). It also has implications for how the international professional organizations, such as the International Council on Social Welfare, the International Association of Schools of Social Work, the International Federation of Social Workers, the International Council of Nursing, the International Association of Social Educators and the International Union of Psychological Science construct ethical documents, how they engage in human rights action, advocacy at the United Nations and with national and regional governments, and so on. Indeed, it may be expected that the confidence to undertake such actions is enhanced by an appropriate sense of cultural humility, acceptance, dialogue, openness and understanding. So, in the final chapter this discussion turns to a consideration of the way in which this can be constructed and the principal obstacles to its achievement.

10 Embracing diversity

Shared humanity and cultural difference?

Paradox and pluralism in professional values and ethics

This book has examined the relationship between culture, values and ethics in social work and human services. Chapters 1 and 2 argue that the development of social work and human services theories and practices are related to the core concerns of human life. They also explore the ways in which the social phenomena that are the focus of social work and human services are grounded in human cultures. From this, in Chapter 3, it is shown that questions of culture must be taken seriously in looking at the ways in which wider social values provide the ground on which professionalization of these occupations has occurred. In particular, the ethics of these professions are central to the project of professionalization, in the construction of goals (ends) and methods of intervention (means). However, it is noted that this in turn raises questions about how the cultural basis of values underpins this historical development, because the relationship between ends and means reflects particular views about what is good in human lives. So, in Chapters 4 and 5 respectively, the competing arguments for universalist and cultural relativist approaches to professional values and ethics are examined. This discussion then leads in Chapter 6 into a consideration of ethical pluralism as an approach that seeks to move beyond the binary arguments that follow from the distinction between universalism and relativism. Two important areas of human society that have an impact on debates about culture, values and ethics are then explored in Chapter 7 (religion and spirituality) and Chapter 8 (politics), drawing out the relevance of these for thinking about social work and human services ethics in practice and policy.

Chapter 9 begins to summarize these debates and to set out some implications of a pluralistic approach. Most particularly, a paradox is identified at the heart of thinking about culture, values and ethics in these fields, which can be summarized in the following way: while they are central to the achievement of the values of each community, claims to difference (for example in separate social welfare provision) are self-limiting in the same way that claims to individual freedom are self-limiting. The latter, which enables people as individuals and as members of families and communities to exercise independence of thought and choice that are the markers of freedom, is only achievable to the extent that a society is ordered in such a way as to make this possible. Where a society does not sustain such freedom, the claim to cultural diversity is also not sustained. In other words, it is not possible to understand an individual human life taken out of a social context. So, too, it is not possible to understand the claims of culture as the basis of values unless differences are recognized, both between cultures and (just as importantly) *within* cultures. Intercultural relationships may be between nation states, in the international arena or they may be internal to states in the form of multicultural societies. Variations at the level of smaller groups and individuals then add to the complexity.

The implication of these conclusions for social work and human services is that skills, theories and ethics must all take account of such differences and cannot reasonably be constructed in monolithic ways. Ironically, the individuation that is inherent in some theory and practice would appear to allow for this, especially in the way it appears in the tradition of understanding the 'person in their social context' (Green & McDermott, 2010). However, as noted in previous chapters, this has often come to be constructed in ways that imply single explanatory perspectives and do not allow for differentiation in practice. Similarly, collectivist theories have grasped the ways in which values are located in community identity and experience, but they have not always taken account of the ways in which individuals or smaller groups within communities might differ from the dominant social values or between each other.

In a review of social work and human services ethics, Briskman and Noble (1999) ask whether the profession is 'embracing diversity'. While they largely suggest that it is not, they identify one positive development (as of 1999), in the form of the bicultural approach to the Aotearoa-New Zealand Association of Social Workers' code of ethics (the more recent version of which is addressed in Chapter 9). The implication of their argument is that in all aspects of professional values and ethics a more conscious effort must be made to address cultural diversity explicitly. Furthermore, rather than making modest adjustments to thinking or to documents, social work and human services should consciously engage with the task of making the acceptance of diversity a primary value in itself. Briskman and Noble's conclusion is that unless this is done, these professions will not live up to the other primary values that they assert. They suggest that professional ethics should be constructed around the continual review and negotiation of moral understanding. At the same time, they acknowledge that there is a collective dimension to professional ethics that must also be acknowledged, so that the processes of ethical attention to diversity must hold this in tension (Briskman & Noble, 1999, pp. 66–67; compare with: Ross, 2008; Yan, 2008). The process of understanding ethics in cultural context does not occur at the level of 'autonomous' individuals acting in isolation from their memberships of particular social groups (including communities and professions).

This last point rests on a continuing recognition that claims to social justice as a core value usually cut across cultural differences and continue to draw on modernist ideas about how the world 'ought to be' (Reisch, 2002, 2008; Bisman, 2004; Ferguson, 2008; Solas, 2008). Indeed, arguments that members of ethnic minorities, women, people with disabilities, young people, older people, people of different sexualities and so on, all should be recognized in the shaping of social work and human services values and ethics are claims to the idea of social justice. As Reisch (2008) notes in relation to 'race' and culture, this concept seeks equal access for all people to the benefits of a society, irrespective of their specific identities. It is at this point that the different dynamics of social justice and human rights as values become reconciled, in that the claim to equal access and equal opportunity rest on the recognition of the common humanity in each person. In all our differences, which are important to understanding who we are, we are all human beings and therefore should be treated with respect, which includes having our unique characteristics recognized and valued.

Yet this conclusion then leads a pluralist analysis into a further debate about the way in which the claim to the underlying, common view of humanity in all people can sit uncomfortably with the recognition of diversity. It is to this problem that the discussion now turns.

Shared humanity

In a recent discussion of human rights in social work and human services practices, Ife (2009) argues that the risk of strongly held primary values is that they can easily become an inflexible form of universalism, in which a single view of what it is to be human can become imposed by those with power (whether political, economic, professional, academic or cultural). This can lead to an ironic situation in which human rights become associated with totalitarian ways of imposing particular ideals, through asserting that what it is to be human has to take one particular form. The answer, for Ife (2009, p. 130), is to seek a 'shared humanity', in which all members of a community are able to play active roles in the construction of what humanity means, and allows for these definitions to differ and to overlap without having to be identical. This requires that practitioners rethink their understanding of community, in which there is a balance between what unites people and the many differences between them (p. 131).

Webb (2009) argues that Reichert (2003) and Ife (2008) overstate the claims of difference and diversity in relation to human rights (although his main target is Moonie *et al.*, 2004). For Webb, claims to principles such as human rights and social justice can only rest on a very strong form of acknowledging those things that all people share. This Webb (2009, p. 311) unambiguously calls 'sameness'. This is partly a complaint about what he sees as the tendency of social work and human services in recent times to address ideas of human rights and social justice overwhelmingly in terms of what divides people rather than those things that they share. In its most simple terms, Webb's argument is that common or shared ideas about what it is to be human are foundational to claims about rights and justice and any questions about difference and diversity can only be seen as secondary (although at times he gives the appearance of wanting to dispense with these latter ideas altogether). Webb does not address this distinction in such terms, but this is a type of pluralist argument. However, because he does not consider the point explicitly, he then reaches a conclusion that surprisingly appears to wish to jettison the principle of human rights as irredeemably relativist. His argument appears in this sense to ignore the way in which this discourse is based on claims to 'being human', which must have a shared or common view of humanity at their foundation. That is, such claims tend to be universalist and are often criticized as such. In contrast, the argument of this book is that, seen in pluralist terms, both human rights and social justice must be approached at the primary (what we can share) and secondary (what may differentiate us) levels of values. That requires engagement with the messy, difficult and often contradictory demands of practice.

Nussbaum's version of the 'capabilities approach', discussed in Chapter 4, may offer social work and human services a way of thinking in pluralist terms about the core values that are shared between the professions and diverse societies. One of the key aspects of Nussbaum's (2000, pp. 74–86) defence of her approach is that the list of human capabilities that she has developed came from the work she undertook with women's groups in regional India. In other words, she makes the claim that these are 'bottom up' ideas that are widely shared around the world, not simply the impositions of an American academic lawyer and philosopher. Moreover, Nussbaum (2002, pp. 132–133) also asserts that her list is open to critique, debate and reformulation – although she considers it robust precisely because of its multicultural origins. These capabilities are not detailed specifications of what people should have, for example in the sense of stating exactly what a family should look like. They are ways of understanding the basis on which all people might have the sort of opportunities that Ife (2009) is suggesting every person needs in order to be a more active citizen contributing to the continual process of defining and redefining community values.

In this sense, Nussbaum's (2000) list of capabilities (life of normal length; bodily health and integrity; senses, imagination and thought; emotions; practical reason; affiliation; relationship to other species; play; and control over one's environment) are not ends in themselves but means to the many and differing ends which people choose on the basis of their own values. Social work and human services may seek to promote these capabilities, for example in the provision of support and protection for women and children who are subject to family and domestic violence, or assistance for those people with disabilities or older people who need help in daily life but who do not have other sources of care. The actual form of the interventions and services that are developed do not have to follow any one specific pattern, even though they are seeking the same (or common, or shared) ends. Indeed, the extent to which they can take different forms is an indicator of the way in which a society can promote freedom as a primary value. So, to take services for older people as a specific instance, this can best be achieved by having a range of possibilities in which people can receive assistance that most addresses their values. Such options would include support for families providing care and services that substitute for family care; it would also include helping some people to remain in their own homes while giving others the opportunity for various types of supported accommodation, with the latter having the potential to respond appropriately to cultural differences. Clearly providing a range of services in this way then in turn depends on wider social and political commitment to developing appropriate policies and providing resources. This then points to the way in social work and human services also have roles in policy development and advocacy, not only in the actual provision of direct services.

So, is the distinction between 'common' and 'shared' simply semantic, or is there more to it than this? The answer to this question has to be found in the implications of Nussbaum's (2000) and Ife's (2009) constructions of 'humanity' and of 'rights'. Nussbaum's purpose is to identify those aspects of the ways in which people think of a decent life that apply across cultures and so may be said to indicate something about 'being human'. These are the aspects of life that people generally expect to experience, because they are the intrinsic requirements for anyone to live a good human life – such as not living in fear of being assaulted in one's home by one's spouse (Hugman, 2008, p. 128).

In contrast, Ife is seeking to argue for a model of *practice* for social work and human services, in which people are enabled to pursue their own visions of what is good in life, within their everyday family and community relationships. He argues that this would be a gain over those practices in which human rights are defined by reference to a single universal notion of humanity. So it not only avoids imposing an 'expert' definition of humanity 'from above' but also promotes the goal of enabling people to play an active role in understanding and shaping their own lives (Ife, 2009, p. 130).

Yet this is also a goal claimed by Nussbaum (2000, pp. 74–77), who states that she is seeking to find the minimum commonality necessary to be able to speak across cultures while still maintaining the possibility of people within each cultural community defining their own vision of a good life. In this sense, it appears that Nussbaum and Ife are proposing quite similar objectives, in deriving the basis for all cultural communities to be able to pursue their values while protecting individuals and subgroups from oppressions within their communities.

Both Nussbaum (2000, pp. 73–74) and Ife (pp. 129–130) also recognize that too great a focus on difference can lead to exclusionary practices, which can become discrimination and divisiveness. It is this risk against which much recent argument about anti-racism and anti-oppressive practice in social work and human services has argued (Dominelli, 2008; Clifford & Burke, 2009). However, it is here that their arguments seem to part company. For Nussbaum the greater risk is that too great a focus on difference leads to arguments for the supremacy of particular cultures, or aspects of cultures. In this way, she notes (2000, *passim*) that across many cultures women become subordinated through this type of argument. There is a considerable risk that differentiation can create grounds for oppression if members of particular ethnic communities, or women, or other social categories, come to be seen as not fully human. So seeking commonality is the crucial task. Ife too is concerned that discriminations based on 'discourses of difference' (2009, p. 129) can lead to different forms of oppression. However, for him it appears the greater risk is in the imposition of particular views of the good human life, and so prioritizing difference is the imperative. It is this contrast of concerns that lies behind the potential debate between whether it is more helpful to think in terms of 'common' or 'shared' values. In turn, these positions then appear to give priority to universal and relative views of values respectively, even though both Nussbaum and Ife can also be said to have the same underlying concern to find an appropriate balance between that which applies to all people and that which is culturally specific.

Pluralism and ethical conversation

Holding the tension between universality and differentiation in understanding human needs and values requires a pluralistic response. Ethical or value pluralism seeks to find ways of achieving dialogue between different visions of 'the good' (what moral philosophers call 'goods'), rather than arriving at a single unitary position, as discussed in Chapter 6. Such a conversation must be entered into for the sake of finding that which is common or shared and how people can live with differences, not with the intention of 'winning the argument' (Hugman, 2005, p. 129). To recap, primary goods and values are those that can be said to be encountered in most, if not all, societies – they go beyond the biological, for example the need for water, food and shelter, in that they may also include psychological and social factors, such as the need for relationships. Thus, Kekes (1993, p. 42) argues that the primary values can be seen as 'self, intimacy and social order'. Secondary values, such as the particular expectations of selfhood, or what a family should look like, or how a community should be structured, are the ways in which each culture has developed the means to achieve the primary goods. Nussbaum's (2000) list of capabilities can be seen as elaborations of these same notions. Nevertheless, these analysts are agreed that the list of primary goods, and hence primary values, is very short. Although Kekes (1993, p. 43) goes on to say that many secondary values extend and enrich the range of human possibilities (such as those of occupation or profession, talents, competition and solidarity, honour, comfort, privacy), these follow from primary values and must be understood as particular expressions of them in a given context. Not all of these secondary values will be encountered in a specific culture (for example, not every culture has the same understanding of 'privacy' and some languages even do not have an equivalent word).

From this account of pluralism, it may be concluded that professional social work and human services can be seen as part of the means by which modern societies pursue the primary values of self, intimacy and social order. At the same time, the form taken by social work and human services is secondary, as the concrete issues and problems with which practitioners are engaged are encountered and must be resolved at the secondary level of values. So, to use again the example of family violence, this affects the selfhood of each member of the family, it affects the intimate relationships of the family and it also concerns the way in which community norms may be seen to be affected. The same may be said about the neglect or injury of children, the way in which families are assisted in supporting those members who require particular care or assistance, how people who commit offences against others are dealt with and so on.

This pluralistic view of what is common or shared and what is different provides a basis for social work and human services practitioners to consider variations within cultures as well as cross-cultural dialogue. The initial question of how a particular person, family or community understands its values can be addressed not by asking about the secondary values of the dominant culture, such as might be found in formal legal definitions of a family, but of seeking to understand the way in which *these people* in *this situation* understand and express such ideas. Making this sort of concern the basis of cross-cultural practice suggests a more sensitive and flexible approach than a more technocratic view of cultural 'competence' (Dean, 2001; O'Hagan, 2001). This becomes possible when practice draws on the common or shared values of self, intimacy and social order as a starting point for inter-cultural empathy (compare with Nussbaum, 2000, pp. 72, 74). So, for example, the detail of attending to people's names including spelling and pronunciation should be seen as an ethical matter, because it affirms respect for a person's self and their agency, as well as having the practical benefit of establishing better communication.

Holding the tension between a common view of what it is to be human and seeing this question as entirely relative to culture also has great importance for professional ethics. If, as has been argued elsewhere in this book, professions and the societies of which they are part have to reach a point where ethical stances are declared (such as a profession regards social justice as a primary value, or a society states that the ill-treatment of children is unacceptable) then there is very little scope for individuals or groups within these collective entities to simply assert a different position. This is the practical implication of the limitation of freedom that has been discussed above. If the social work and human services professions are to take a pluralist approach to ethics seriously then there need to be other ways in which differences can be embraced rather than simply tolerated in an assumption that principles such as human rights and social justice will always achieve this. A pluralist approach can only succeed in conditions of an open dialogue, where the goal is to listen and to share values, on the basis of those things that can be agreed as common to humanity. However, before concluding the discussion by summarizing the implications of this for professional ethics, there is another potential barrier that must be addressed, that of the way in which even those values that are widely held as primary to a profession can prevent alternative views being expressed.

The challenge of 'fundamentalisms'

Midgley and Sanzenbach (1989) examine the phenomenon of 'fundamentalism' in religion and its implications for social work and human services. They are very careful to note that this is a concern with a particular approach to religion and not to religion overall, which they describe in detail as also having had a progressive role in the development of social work and human services (compare with Chapter 7). Nor do they confine their analysis to a particular religion, as they note that all the major world faiths have fundamentalist groups or streams within them. Thus, it is not that social work and human services values are incompatible with religious belief, as there are many arguments showing the close connections and acknowledging the ways in which these professions often developed out of religious ideals (1989, pp. 274–275, p. 280).

The characteristics of fundamentalism that Midgley and Sanzenbach identify derive from a concern to promote a singular understanding of 'truth', often based on a literal reading of religious texts and in which tradition is the central criterion for determining what is true (1989, p. 278). In religious fundamentalism this is most usually an attempt to deny or counter the impact on systems of belief of the very sorts of social change that have led to the professionalization of social work and human services. This struggle to resist the impact of modernity then leads to a position that is 'dogmatic and intolerant of dissent' (ibid.).

It is this last aspect of fundamentalism that is of broader relevance to values and ethics in social work and human services. One problem that has been discussed in previous chapters is how appropriate responses can be made to people in those communities whose values are defined in terms of traditional beliefs that appear dogmatic. Where services are voluntary, this can be seen as plausible in terms of professional ethics, because it can be seen in terms of people acting on the basis of human agency. Professional ethics can even support arguments for culturally relevant separate services on such grounds. The problem arises in situations of involuntary services, such as those with protective or corrective functions. In such situations, legal requirements provide the basis for making practice decisions in which those who are the subjects of interventions may not voluntarily choose them – although there is always the necessity of acting with as much cultural sensitivity as is possible.

But what of other value positions that are dogmatic and intolerant of dissent? Ife (2010) questions the approach taken to human rights as an example of secular fundamentalism. He argues that the view of human rights as 'natural' led to the formulation of statements of human rights as political and legal documents such as the *Universal Declaration of Human Rights* (UN, 1948) and the various other more focused declarations and conventions that follow from it (regarding women, children, disabled people, Indigenous people and so on). However, for Ife, this then causes statements of rights, which are historical constructs, to be accorded the standing of immutable truths: 'they no longer need to be questioned, but must be accepted and implemented' (2010, p. 153). From this conclusion, Ife then criticizes approaches to human rights that do not allow for debate, disagreement and dissent as 'fundamentalist' (p. 155).

Asad (2000) has questioned the inherent legalism in the pursuit of human rights as an often overly thin concept, because a legal model requires someone to be able to make a claim against an agent who has the responsibility to make some redress. Not everyone may have access to law in this way. Moreover, not all violations of a person's humanity occur in contexts where a legalistic model is relevant. For example, within families recourse to law often signals the breakdown of relationships and the same can be said also of community relationships. As Asad notes (2000, section 51), human relationships more often require values of 'compassion, patience, commitment, selflessness, etc.'. For social work and human services, in which human rights together with social justice are asserted as a primary value, this critique presents an important challenge.

Yet, the alternative that Ife proposes, an inductive construction of rights 'from below' actually appears to resemble the methods used by Nussbaum (2000) in formulating her list of human capabilities, namely by working with people in context and listening to their values and visions of a good human life. It is also the case that when approached in this way, documents such as the *Universal Declaration* and other UN instruments can become powerful tools in the hands of people who otherwise lack power to challenge oppressions and violations. Where social workers and other human services practitioners act as allies with people whose rights have been violated, to make use of both quasi-legal and other means of seeking resolution, the human rights and social justice discourses can be very powerful. For example, work undertaken by Australian social workers with the United Nations High Commission for Refugees (UNHCR) contributes to the greater recognition of the endemic problem of rape and sexual assault of women and girls in refugee situations (Pittaway *et al.*, 2007). Such work contributes to the wider debates about rape as a crime against humanity and as a war crime (Zawati, 2007).

Such a debate points to the importance of social work and human services avoiding value positions that can be described as 'fundamentalist'. This is the case whether these are religious or secular, or are promoting dogmatic and intolerant views concerning even the primary values that are claimed in professional ethics. It must also be noted that not every defence, or criticism, of either universalist or relativist positions on professional ethics is to be seen as dogmatic or intolerant. What is at issue here is the willingness to consider different views and to be able to debate and defend ideas, with the view always to ensuring that change and development are possible through recognizing and embracing diversity.

Conclusion: celebrating difference and embracing diversity together

This book has presented an argument for a pluralist approach to thinking about culture, values and ethics in social work and human services. To recap, pluralism assumes that there are many ways of thinking about values and ethics that may be reasonable. It is not only that different approaches ask different questions (although this is the case) but also that in doing so the values that are held may be inconsistent with each other (Hinman, 2008, pp. 52–54; compare with Nagel, 1979). In addition, as well as inconsistency and incompatibility, there are even times when values are simply not comparable with each other, either because it cannot be said which is 'better' or because they are of such different qualities that comparison is totally impossible (Kekes, 1993; Chang, 1997).

One of the ways of addressing such pluralities of value is in recognizing that they may actually have a contextualized relevance (Chang, 1997). For example, the debate noted above regarding human rights as a culturally grounded, Western construct, often fails to consider that the human rights and social justice discourses have frequently proven very effective in the public arena when considering relationships at a macro level in many different cultural contexts. However, at the level of family, and sometimes small-scale community relationships, to speak of human rights and social justice may not make the same sense as these values appear to depersonalize those things that across many cultures are intrinsically personal (Yip, 2004; Ross, 2008; Yan, 2008). The biggest problem lies in the middle ground, for example in debates about the relevance of such values for micro-level professional practices (including counselling, casework and service provision), where these concern 'the personal' but are also to some extent in the 'public domain' in so far as they involve professionals and human service agencies. The pluralist position does not provide an easy answer for this, but suggests that dialogue around these questions must be engaged in, accepting that agreements will often be provisional. The objective is 'sufficient' rather than 'incontrovertible' sharing of values and goals.

A crucial dimension of the ethical pluralist approach is to question dichotomies and statements that advocate an 'essentialized' view of any value or facet of human life (Sewpaul, 2007). 'Essentialized' here includes overarching generalities, such as 'African values', 'Asian values', 'Western values' and so on. As Sewpaul suggests, and the above argument has endorsed, to speak of such concepts in monolithic ways ignores the many 'historical tensions and contradictions' that are found in any of these broad constructs (Sewpaul, 2007, p. 402). While the resulting dichotomy of the 'West-against-the-rest' has some historical validity, in terms of the institutional origins of professionalization in social work and human services (see Chapter 3, also: Healy, 2008; Hugman, 2010), it oversimplifies the relationships between and within national and cultural groupings. As Sewpaul (2007, pp. 403–404) argues:

> We must be careful about reifying and idealizing Asian culture based on collectivism, respect for family, and as embodying unifying and holistic principles and intuitive functioning as opposed to Western culture which is represented as fragmented, individualised and reductionistic.

In so far as it has any use at all, such a dichotomy only achieves certain goals, such as in highlighting the importance of understanding key historical factors in debates about the nature of social work and human services as professional practices and structures. It does not explain everything that is necessary to grasp the complex picture.

Arguments that the aims of 'cross-cultural competence' are oversimplified come from the same critique (Dean, 2001; O'Hagan, 2001; Weaver, 2004). Recognition of cultural diversity requires attention to the (potential) differences of values in respect of all the aspects of human life with which social work and human services are concerned. This process cannot be confined to technical approaches in developing appropriate responses to such differences, but is more often developed through critical ways of integrating theory with practice that are variously called 'reflexive practice' or 'praxis' (see, for example, Healy, 2005). This way of understanding the relationship between theories and practices sees them as interactive and so continually developing.

This means that knowledge, skills and values that are helpful in working more effectively in multicultural practice are not fixed but should be seen as growing and changing as practitioners engage self-critically with their own practices. At the same time, the need for awareness, sensitivity and flexibility that is called for in a multicultural view of social work and human services has to be made explicit so that new entrants to these professions can be enabled to develop these capacities and existing members can be encouraged to engage more consciously with the difficult work of sustaining them. So the educational and training programmes in these fields, including life-long continuing education, must also be expected to provide the basis for individual practitioners to be equipped to engage actively in these processes.

From a comparative study of occupational therapy students in Aotearoa-New Zealand and Canada, Forwell *et al.* (2001, p. 101) noted the following wisdom from one of the students: '[y]ou have got to feel good about yourself and your culture before you start to feel good about others'. This does not mean that it is helpful to ignore those things about one's own culture that can and should be criticized thoroughly. But a critical perspective does not mean having to be negative about everything; all cultures have aspects that their members would wish to celebrate and even share with others, as well as those things 'we would be better off without' (Rorty, 1999, p. 276). What it does mean is that unless social workers and other human services professionals are able to articulate an understanding of the differences between those aspects of culture that may be celebrated and those that should be jettisoned, to recognize that others are likely to disagree with the choices made and not to be disillusioned by this, then the capacity to work in multicultural contexts is likely to be quite limited.

The implication of a pluralist perspective is that because of the inconsistencies, incompatibilities and incomparabilities between values, a uniform agreement is highly unlikely, not only at the global level but also even within a specific culture. This means that practitioners, both as individuals and in the form of collectivities such as professional associations and unions, must be prepared to engage in the necessary dialogues about values, both within these professions and with people in their surrounding societies. It is widely observed that, notwithstanding the differences that pluralism presumes, there will be some underlying points of connection in which all those parties to the conversation will know and agree that they are talking about 'social work and human services' (compare: Healy, 2005; Sewpaul, 2007; Dominelli, 2008; Ferguson, 2008; Clifford & Burke, 2009). In some way, each strand within social work and human services theory and practice is directed towards social change and can concur that there are some things that simply cannot be defended on any cultural grounds. What differs is the way in which various value positions understand the causes of and resolutions to the issues and problems with which social work and human services are concerned, including the focus of intervention (between the micro, mezzo and macro levels of individuals, families, groups, communities, research and policy). Beyond that, the cultural points of reference for affirming or rejecting particular values mean that within as well as outside these professions there is considerable diversity.

So, social work and human services are left with a contradiction that has to be encountered and actively addressed. To summarize, the core professional values of human rights and social justice rest on the idea that 'what it is to be human' is shared in common by all people. It is the idea that all people must be treated as fully human that gives these principles their moral force. Yet, at the same time, a multicultural world requires careful attention to cultural differences; these differences even include varying positions on the values of human rights and social justice (especially the former) and how these relate to specific cultural practices. Cultural differences are encountered in every aspect of social work and human services practice, in the meaning of a wide variety of personal and social problems and issues – in families, in communities and in the wider social and economic life of a country. If social work and human services professionals are to work with this contradiction it has to be identified, grasped and constantly rethought through critical and reflexive practice. The pluralist approach suggests that the aim is not to overcome this challenge, as such a goal would assume that the differences between cultural values had somehow been removed or transcended. Instead it points to the inevitable task of understanding ('self' as well as 'other') and responding in ways that embody a wide range of the values that are claimed by more specific discussions of professional ethics, such as respect, honesty and integrity.

What, then, are the implications for formal statements of professional ethics that have been identified above as key features of modern professions? As has been discussed in this chapter and in previous chapters, this analysis first indicates that it is both necessary and possible for statements and codes to address cultural diversity of values. This can be done in several ways, including the inclusion of the recognition of cultural diversity and commitments to addressing this and in identifying particular groups who have a claim to overt recognition (such as in the bicultural code of ethics in Aotearoa-New Zealand – ANZASW, 2008). Such measures are not to be regarded as a panacea in which the challenges of cultural diversity are somehow smoothed away, but as ways in which members of these professions from diverse backgrounds can engage in dialogue and seek to develop practices that are more relevant for multicultural societies.

It is also the case that cultural pluralism cannot be divorced from ethical pluralism. The former is the claim that cultures may reasonably differ in those things that are valued; the latter is the argument that different ethical principles may reasonably be used to understand questions of values and to provide the basis for action. So, just as practice in social work and human services has to find ways of addressing the common shared humanity lived in diverse ways in different cultures, so too it has to be grounded in an ethics that is capable of holding together the debates between moral duties, consequences, virtues, care, the natural world and other ethical approaches (Hugman, 2005).

At a more general level, it can be observed that debates about culture and values in relation to professional ethics can be avoided by some members of these professions for a whole variety of reasons – because they appear irresolvable, they generate strong feelings, it is possible to cause offence or make mistakes, or even that such issues are seen as better addressed through political structures. As has been argued in various places throughout this discussion, each of these concerns is misplaced, however understandable, because they prevent social work and human services from engaging with a crucial aspect of the contemporary world, that of a diversity of cultures with the resulting competition of values. Instead, the argument here has been that these professions should celebrate difference as a vital aspect of 'what it is to be human' and embrace diversity in the ways in which social work and human services knowledge, skills and values are constructed as a messy, unpredictable and therefore challenging but nevertheless shared activity.

Bibliography

Addams, J. (2002 [1907]) *Democracy and Social Ethics*. Ed. Siegfreid, C. H. Urbana and Chicago, University of Illinois Press.

Akutsu, P. D., Castillo, E. D. & Snowden, L. R. (2007) 'Differential referral patterns to ethnic-specific and mainstream mental health programs for four Asian American groups', *American Journal of Orthopsychiatry*, 77(1), pp. 95–103.

Allen, I., Hogg, D. & Peace, S. (1992) *Elderly People: Choice, Participation and Satisfaction*. London, Policy Studies Institute.

Altham, J. E. J. (1995) 'Reflection and confidence', in Altham, J. E. J. & Harrison, R. (eds) *World, Mind, and Ethics*. Cambridge, Cambridge University Press.

Annan, K. (1997) 'Ignorance not knowledge ... makes enemies of man', *UNHCRH*. Electronic document, downloaded on 21 September 2010 from www.unhchr.ch/huricane/huricane.nsf/view01/EF16892B9B9D46ABC125662E00352F63?opendocument.

Anti-Slavery Society (2008) *Fighting Slavery Today*. Electronic document, downloaded on 8 August 2011 from www.anti-slaverysociety.addr.com/tocslavery.htm.

Aotearoa-New Zealand Association of Social Workers [ANZASW] (2008) *Code of Ethics*. Christchurch, ANZASW.

Asad, T. (2000) 'What do human rights do? An anthropological inquiry', *Theory & Event*, 4(4). Electronic document, downloaded on 25 May 2007 from http://muse.jhu.edu/journals/theory_and_event/v004/4.4asad.html.

Asai, M. O. & Kameoka, V. A. (2005) 'The influence of *sekentei* on family caregiving and underutilization of social services among Japanese caregivers', *Social Work*, 50(2), pp. 111–118.

Australian Association of Social Workers [AASW] (2010) *Code of Ethics*. Barton ACT, AASW.

Australian Institute of Welfare and Community Workers [AIWCW] (2010) *Who Is A Community Worker?* Electronic document, downloaded on 2 February 2011 from www.aiwcw.org.au/content/who-community-worker.

Azmi, S. (1997) 'Professionalism and social diversity' in Hugman, R., Peelo, M. & Soothill, K. (eds) *Concepts of Care: Developments in Health and Social Welfare*. London, Arnold.

Baines, D. (2008) 'Race, resistance, and restructuring: emerging skills in the new social services', *Social Work*, 53(2), pp. 123–131.

Baldry, E. (2010) 'Mental health disorders and cognitive disability in the criminal justice system', keynote address to the *Community Legal Centres NSW Conference*, Sydney, 6 May.

Banks, S. (2004) *Ethics, Accountability and the Social Professions*. Basingstoke, Palgrave-Macmillan.

Banks, S. (2006) *Ethics and Values in Social Work*. Basingstoke, Palgrave-Macmillan.

Banks, S. (ed.) (2010) *Ethical Issues in Youth Work*. 2nd Edition. London, Routledge.

Banks, S. & Gallagher, A. (2009) *Ethics in Professional Life: Virtues in Health and Social Care*. Basingstoke, Palgrave-Macmillan.

Banks, S. & Imam, U. (2000) 'Principles, rules and qualities: an ethical framework for youth work', *International Journal of Adolescence and Youth*, 9(1), pp. 65–82.

Banks, S. & Nøhr, K. (2003) *Teaching Practical Ethics for the Social Professions*. Copenhagen, FESET.

Banks, S. & Nøhr, K. (eds) (2011) *Practising Social Work Ethics Around the World: Cases and Commentaries*. London, Taylor & Francis.

Barbarin, O. A. (2003) 'Social risks and child development in South Africa: a nation's program to protect the human rights of children', *American Journal of Orthopsychiatry*, 73(3), pp. 248–254.

Barn, R. (2007) '"Race", ethnicity and child welfare: a fine balancing act', *British Journal of Social Work*, 37(8), pp. 1425–1434.

Barsky, A. E. (2009) *Ethics and Values in Social Work: an Integrated Approach for a Comprehensive Curriculum*. New York, Oxford University Press.

Barth, F. (1998 [1969]) *Ethnic Groups and Boundaries: the Social Organization of Cultural Difference*. Long Grove IL, Waveland Press.

Basu, R., Basu, A. & Kesselman, M. (1978) 'Racism, classism and welfare', *Catalyst*, 1(3), pp. 24–35.

Bauman, Z. (1993) *Postmodern Ethics*. Oxford, Basil Blackwell.

Bauman, Z. (1994) *Alone Again: Ethics After the Age of Certainty*. London, Demos.

Bauman, Z. (1995) *Life in Fragments*. Oxford, Basil Blackwell.

Bauman, Z. (2001a) *The Individualized Society*. Cambridge, Polity Press.

Bauman, Z. (2001b) 'Whatever happened to compassion?', in Bentley, T. & Stedman-Jones, D. (eds) *The Moral Universe*. London, Demos.

Baxter, J. E. (2005) *The Archaeology of Childhood: Children, Gender and Material Culture*. Walnut Creek CA, AltaMira Press.

BBC (2011) 'Women in veils detained as France enforces ban', *BBC News Europe*. Electronic document, downloaded 1 August 2011 from www.bbc. co.uk/news/world-europe-13031397.

Beauchamp, T. L. & Childress, J. F. (2009) *Principles of Biomedical Ethics*, 6th Edition. New York, Oxford University Press.

Beckett, C. & Maynard, A. (2005) *Values and Ethics in Social Work: an Introduction*. London, Sage.

Bell, D. A. & Bauer, J. R. (eds) (1999) *The East Asian Challenge for Human Rights*. New York, Cambridge University Press.

Benedict, R. (2005 [1934]) *Patterns of Culture*. New York, Mariner Books.

Benhabib, S. (2002) *The Claims of Culture*. Princeton NJ, Princeton University Press.

Benhabib, S. (2004) *The Rights of Others*. New York, Cambridge University Press.

Benhabib, S. (2006) *Another Cosmopolitanism: Hospitality, Sovereignty and Democratic Iterations*. New York, Oxford University Press.

Bentham, J. (1970 [1781]) *An Introduction to the Principles of Morals and Legislation*. London, Athlone Press.

Beresford, P. (2000) 'Service users' knowledges and social work theory: conflict or collaboration', *British Journal of Social Work*, 30(4), pp. 489–503.

Beresford, P. (2003) *It's Our Lives: A Short Theory of Knowledge, Distance and Experience*. London, Open Services Project.

Berger, P. (2004) *Questions of Faith: a Skeptical Affirmation of Christianity*. Oxford, Blackwell Publishing.

Berlin, I. (1969) *Four Essays on Liberty*. Oxford, Oxford University Press.

Berlin, I. (1992) *The Crooked Timber of Humanity: Chapters in the History of Ideas*. Ed. Hardy, H. New York, Vintage Books.

Biestek, F. P. (1957) *The Casework Relationship*. Chicago, Loyola University Press.

Board of Inquiry into the Protection of Aboriginal Children from Sexual Abuse [BIPACSA] (2007) *Ampe Akelyernemane Meke Mekarle: 'Little Children are Sacred'*. Darwin, Northern Territory Government.

Bisman, C. (2004) 'Social work values: the moral core of the profession', *British Journal of Social Work*, 34(1), pp. 109–123.

Blackstock, C. (2004) *Keeping the Promise: the Convention on the Rights of the Child and the Lived Experiences of First Nations Children and Youth*. Ottawa, First Nations Child and Family Caring Society of Canada.

Blackstock, C. & Trocmé, (2005) 'Community-based child welfare for Aboriginal children: supporting resilience through structural change', *Social Policy Journal of New Zealand*, 24, pp. 12–33.

Blom-Cooper, L. J. (1985) *A Child in Trust*. London, Brent Health Authority.

Bondi, L., Carr, D., Clark, C. & Clegg, C. (eds) (2011) *Towards Practice Wisdom*. Farnham, Ashgate.

Borelli, K. (1975) 'The implications of the new ethnicity for American social work', *International Social Work*, 18(1), pp. 1–9.

Bowles, W., Collingridge, M., Curry, S. & Valentine, B. (2006) *Ethical Practice in Social Work: an Applied Approach*. Crows Nest NSW, Allen & Unwin.

Bowpitt, G. (1998) 'Evangelical Christianity, secular Humanism and the genesis of British social work', *British Journal of Social Work*, 28(5), pp. 675–693.

Brandt Commission [The Independent Commission on International Development] (1980) *North-South: a Program for Survival*. London, Pan Books.

Briskman, L. (2007) *Social Work with Indigenous Communities*. Leichhardt NSW, Federation Press.

Briskman, L. & Noble, C. (1999) 'Social work ethics: embracing diversity?', in Pease, B. & Fook, J. (eds) *Transforming Social Work Practice: Critical Postmodern Perspectives*. St Leonards NSW, Allen & Unwin.

Burton, L. A. & DeWolf Bosek, M. S. (2000) 'When religion may be an ethical issue', *Journal of Religion and Health*, 39(2), pp. 97–106.

Butcher, H., Banks, S. & Henderson, P. with Robertson, J. (2007) *Critical Community Practice*. Bristol, Policy Press.

Butrym, Z. (1976) *The Nature of Social Work*. London, Macmillan.

Canda, E. R. & Furman, L. D. (1999) *Spiritual Diversity in Social Work Practice: the Heart of Helping*. New York, The Free Press.

Canadian Association of Social Workers/Association Canadien des Travailleuses et Travaileurs Sociaux [CASW/ACTS] (2005) *Code of Ethics/Code de Déontologie de l'ACTS*. Ottawa, CASW/ACTS.

Carey, M. (2008) 'What difference does it make? Contrasting organization and converging outcomes regarding the privatization of state social work in England and Canada', *International Social Work*, 51(1), pp. 83–94.

Carr-Saunders, A. M. & Wilson, P. A. (1962) *The Professions*. London, Oxford University Press.

Caulk, R. S. (1980) 'Human services planning in the 1980s', *Journal of Alternative Human Services*, 6(1), pp. 29–32.

Centre for Contemporary Cultural Studies (1982) *The Empire Strikes Back: Race and Racism in 70s Britain*. London, Hutchinson & Co.

Chan, R. K. H. & Wang, Y. (2009) 'Controlled decentralization: *minban* education reform in China', *Journal of Comparative Social Welfare*, 25(1), pp. 27–36.

Chang, J., Rhee, S. & Weaver, D. (2006) 'Characteristics of child abuse in immigrant Korean families and correlates of placement decisions', *Child Abuse & Neglect*, 30, pp. 881–891.

Chang, R. (1997) 'Introduction', in Chang, R. (ed.) *Incommensurability, Incompatibility and Practical Reason*. Cambridge MA, Harvard University Press.

Cherniss, J. & Hardy, H. (2010) 'Isaiah Berlin', in Zalta, E. N. (ed.) *The Stanford Encyclopedia of Philosophy (Fall 2010 Edition)*. Electronic document, downloaded on 8 April 2011 from http://plato.stanford.edu/archives/fall2010/entries/berlin.

Chow, J. C. C., Auh, E. Y., Scharlach, A. E., Lehning, A. J. & Goldstein, C. (2010) 'Types and sources of support received by family caregivers of older adults from diverse racial and ethnic groups', *Journal of Ethnic and Cultural Diversity in Social Work*, 19(3), pp. 175–194.

Christie, A. (2010) 'Whiteness and the politics of "race" in the child protection guidelines in Ireland', *European Journal of Social Work*, 13(2), pp. 199–215.

Chui, E. (2007) 'Changing norms and pragmatics of co-residence in east Asian countries', *International Journal of Sociology of the Family*, 33(1), pp. 1–24.

Clark, C. (2000) *Social Work Ethics: Politics, Principles & Practice*. Basingstoke, Macmillan.

Clifford, D. & Burke, B. (2009) *Anti-Oppressive Ethics and Values in Social Work*. Basingstoke, Palgrave-Macmillan.

Cnaan, R. A. & Newman, E. (2010) 'The safety net and faith-based services', *Journal of Religion & Spirituality in Social Work: Social Thought*, 29(4), pp. 321–336.

Colebatch, H. K. (2009) *Policy*. New York, McGraw-Hill.

Congress, E. P. (1999) *Social Work Values and Ethics: Identifying and Resolving Personal Dilemmas*. Chicago, Nelson-Hall.

Congress, E. & McAuliffe, D. (2006) 'Professional ethics: social work codes in Australia and the United States', *International Social Work*, 49(2), pp. 165–176.

Coombe, V. & Little, A. (eds) (1986) *Race and Social Work: a Guide to Training*. London, Routledge.

Corey, G., Corey, M. S. & Callanan, P. (2007) *Issues and Ethics in the Helping Professions*. 7th Edition. Belmont CA, Thomson Brooks/Cole.

Cousée, F., Roets, G. & De Bie, M. (2009) 'Empowering the powerful: challenging hidden processes of marginalization in youth work policy and practice in Belgium', *Critical Social Policy*, 29(3), pp. 421–442.

Cousins, C. (1987) *Controlling Social Welfare*. Brighton, Wheatseaf.

Cox, D. & Pawar, M. (2006) *International Social Work*. London and Los Angeles, Sage Publications.

Cox, P. (2010) 'Juvenile justice reform and policy convergence in the new Vietnam', *Youth Justice*, 10(3), pp. 227–244.

Davies, C. (1996) 'The sociology of professions and the profession of gender', *Sociology*, 39(4), pp. 661–678.

Day, P. J. (2000) *A New History of Social Welfare*. 3rd Edition. Boston MA, Allyn & Bacon.

Dean, R. G. (2001) 'The myth of cross-cultural competence', *Families in Society: the Journal of Contemporary Human Services*, 82(6), pp. 623–630.

Dent, M. (1999) 'Professional judgement and the role of clinical guidelines and evidence-based medicine (EBM): Netherlands, Britain and Sweden', *Journal of Interprofessional Care*, 13(2), pp. 151–164.

Derber, C. (1987) 'Managing professionals: ideological proletarianization and post-industrial labour', *Theory and Society*, 12(3), pp. 309–341.

Dhand, A. (2002) 'The dharma of ethics, the ethics of dharma: quizzing the ideals of Hinduism', *The Journal of Religious Ethics*, 30(3), pp. 347–372.

Dickson, J. (2004) *A Spectator's Guide to World Religions: an Introduction to the Big Five*. Sydney, Blue Bottle Books.

Doe, S. S.-J., Han, H. K. & McCaslin, R. (2009) 'Cultural and ethical issues in Korea's recent elder abuse reporting system', *Journal of Elder Abuse and Neglect*, 21(2), pp. 170–185.

Dominelli, L. (2002) *Anti-Oppressive Social Work Theory and Practice*. Basingstoke, Palgrave-Macmillan.

Dominelli, L. (2008) *Anti-Racist Social Work*. 3rd Edition. Basingstoke, Palgrave-Macmillan.

Dominelli, L. (2010) 'Anti-oppressive ethics', in Gray, M. & Webb, S. A. (eds) *Ethics and Value Perspectives in Social Work*. Basingstoke, Palgrave-Macmillan.

Dominelli, L. & Holloway, M. (2008) 'Ethics and governance in social work research in the UK', *British Journal of Social Work*, 38(5), pp. 1009–1024.

Dominelli, L., Lorenz, W. & Soydan, H. (2001) *Beyond Racial Divides: Ethnicities in Social Work Practice*. Aldershot, Ashgate/Centre for Evaluative and Developmental Research.

Dove, N. (2010) 'A return to traditional health care practices: a Ghanaian study', *Journal of Black Studies*, 40(5), pp. 823–834.

Doyal, L. & Gough, I. (1991) *A Theory of Human Need*. Basingstoke, Macmillan.

Elliott, D. & Segal, U. A. (2008) 'International social work', in Sowers, K. M., White, B. W. & Dulmus, C. N. (eds) *Comprehensive Handbook of Social Work and Social Welfare*. Hoboken NJ, John Wiley & Sons.

England, H. (1983) *Social Work as Art*. London, Allen & Unwin.

Eriksen, T. H. (2006) *Ethnicity and Nationalism*. 2nd Edition. London, Pluto Press.

Etzioni, A. (ed.) (1969) *The Semi-Professions and Their Organization*. Englewood Cliffs NJ, The Free Press.

Evans, T. & Garwick, A. (2002) 'Children with special health care needs', *Journal of Social Work in Disability and Rehabilitation*, 1(2), pp. 7–24.

Faherty, V. E. (2006) 'Social welfare before the Elizabethan Poor Laws: the early Christian tradition, AD 33 to 313', *Journal of Sociology and Social Welfare*, 33(2), pp. 107–122.

Feng, J.-Y., Chen, S.-J., Wilk, N. C., Yang, W.-P. & Fetzer, S. (2009) 'Kindergarten teachers' experience of reporting child abuse in Taiwan: dancing on the edge', *Children and Youth Services Review*, 31(3), pp. 405–409.

Ferguson, I. (2008) *Reclaiming Social Work: Challenging Neo-Liberalism and Promoting Social Justice*. London, Sage Publications.

Ferrarini, T. & Sjöberg, O. (2010) 'Social policy and health: transition countries in a comparative perspective', *International Journal of Social Welfare*, 19, pp. 60–88.

Figueira-McDonough, J. (2007) *The Welfare State and Social Work: Pursuing Social Justice*. Los Angeles, Sage Publications.

Finch, J. (1989) *Family Obligations and Social Change*. Cambridge, Polity Press.

Flaherty, C., Collins-Camargo, C. & Lee, E. (2008) 'Privatization of child welfare services: lessons learned from experienced states regarding site readiness assessment and planning', *Children and Youth Services Review*, 30(7), pp. 809–820.

Fluke, J. D., Yuan, Y. Y. T., Henderson, J. & Curtis, P. A. (2003) 'Disproportionate representation of race and ethnicity in child maltreatment: investigation and victimization', *Children and Youth Services Review*, 25(5/6), pp. 359–373.

Fook, J. (2002) *Social Work: Critical Theory and Practice*. London, Sage Publications.

Forsythe, B. (1995) 'Discrimination in social work – an historical note', *British Journal of Social Work*, 25(1), pp. 1–6.

Forwell, S. J., Whiteford, G. & Dyck, I. (2001) 'Cultural competence in New Zealand and Canada: occupational therapy students' reflections on class and fieldwork curriculum', *The Canadian Journal of Occupational Therapy*, 68(2), pp. 90–103.

Francis, R. D. (2009) *Ethics for Psychologists*. 2nd Edition. Oxford, Blackwell Publishing.

Fraser, N. (2009) 'Social justice in the age of identity politics: redistribution, recognition and participation', in Henderson, G. & Waterstone, M. (eds) *Geographic Thought: a Praxis Perspective*. New York, Routledge.

Freeman, S. J. (2000) *Ethics: an Introduction to Philosophy and Practice*. Belmont, CA, Wadsworth.

Freidson, E. (1983a) 'The theory of professions: state of the art', in Dingwall, R. & Lewis, P. S. C. (eds) *The Sociology of the Professions*. New York, St Martin's Press.

Freidson, E. (1983b) 'The reorganization of the professions by regulation', *Law and Human Behavior'*, 7(2/3), pp. 279–290.

Freidson, E. (1984) 'The changing nature of professional control', *Annual Review of Sociology*, 10(1), pp. 1–20.

Freidson, E. (1994) *Professionalism Reborn: Theory, Prophecy and Policy*. Chicago, University of Chicago Press.

Freidson, E. (2001) *Professionalism: the Third Logic*. Chicago, University of Chicago Press.

Fry, S. T. & Johnstone, M.-J. (2002) *Ethics in Nursing Practice: a Guide to Ethical Decision Making*. 2nd Edition. Oxford, Blackwell Publishing.

Fry, S. T., Veatch, R. M. & Taylor, C. (eds) (2010) *Case Studies in Nursing Ethics*. 4th Edition. Sudbury MA, Jones and Bartlett Publishing.

Furman, L. D., Benson, P. W., Grimwood, C. & Canda, E. (2004) 'Religion and spirituality in social work education and direct practice at the millennium: a survey of UK social workers', *British Journal of Social Work*, 34(6), pp. 767–792.

Gallagher, E. (2004) 'Parents victimised by their children', *Australia and New Zealand Journal of Family Therapy*, 25(1), pp. 1–12.

Gasper, D. (2006) 'Cosmopolitan presumption? On Martha Nussbaum and her commentators', *Development and Change*, 37(6), pp. 1222–1246.

Gauntlett, E., Hugman, R., Kenyon, P. & Logan, P. (2000) *A Meta-Analysis of Prevention and Early Intervention Action. Research Report #11*. Canberra, Australia Government Printing Service.

Gershoff, E. T. (2002) 'Corporal punishment by parents and associated child behaviors and experiences: a meta-analytic and theoretical review', *Psychological Bulletin*, 128(4), pp. 539–579.

Gewirth, A. (1978) *Reason and Morality*. Chicago, University of Chicago Press.

Gilligan, P. (2010) 'Faith based approaches', in Gray, M. & Webb, S. A. (eds) *Ethics and Value Perspectives in Social Work*. Basingstoke, Palgrave-Macmillan.

Gilroy, P. (1987) *There Ain't No Black in the Union Jack*. London, Hutchinson.

Glass, A. P., Chen, L.-K., Hwang, E., Ono, U. & Nahapetyan, L. (2010) 'A cross-cultural comparison of hospice development in Japan, South Korea and Taiwan', *Journal of Cross-Cultural Gerontology*, 25, pp. 1–19.

Gould, N. (1996) 'Social work education and the "crisis of the professions"' in Gould, N. & Taylor, I. (eds) *Reflective Learning for Social Work*. Aldershot, Arena.

Grace, D. (1994) 'Social justice: a new utopianism?' in Wearing, M. & Berreen, R. (eds) *Welfare and Social Policy in Australia*. Sydney, Harcourt Brace.

Graham, J. R. & Shier, M. (2009) 'Religion and social work: an analysis of faith traditions, themes, and global North/South authorship', *Journal of Religion & Spirituality in Social Work*, 28(1), pp. 215–233.

Graham, M. (2002) *Social Work and African-Centred Worldviews*. Birmingham, Venture Press.

Gray, M. (1996) 'Moral theory for social work', *Social Work – Stellenbosch*, 32(4), pp. 289–295.

Gray, M. (2005) 'Dilemmas of international social work: paradoxical processes of indigenization, universalism and imperialism', *International Journal of Social Welfare*, 14, pp. 231–238.

Gray, M. & Fook, J. (2004) 'The quest for a universal social work: some issues and implications', *Social Work Education*, 23(5), pp. 625–644.

Gray, M. & Webb, S. A. (eds) (2010) *Ethics and Value Perspectives in Social Work*. Basingstoke, Palgrave-Macmillan.

Gray, M., Coates, J. & Yellow Bird, M. (eds) (2008) *Indigenous Social Work Around the World: Towards Culturally Relevant Education and Practice*. Aldershot, Ashgate.

Green, D. & McDermott, F. (2010) 'Social work from inside and between complex systems: perspectives on person-in-environment for today's social work', *British Journal of Social Work*, 40(8), pp. 2414–2430.

Green, M. (2010) 'Youth workers as converters? Ethical issues in faith-based youth work', in Banks, S. (ed.) *Ethical Issues in Youth Work*, 2nd Edition. Abingdon, Routledge.

Green, S. & Baldry, E. (2008) 'Building Indigenous Australian social work', *Australian Social Work*, 61(4), pp. 389–402.

Greenwood, E. (1957) 'Attributes of a profession', *Social Work*, 2(3), pp. 44–55.

Gupta, R. (2009) 'Systems perspective: understanding care giving of the elderly in India', *Health Care for Women International*, 30(12), pp. 1040–1054.

Habermas, J. (1990) *Moral Consciousness and Communicative Action*. Trans. Lenhardt, C. & Nicholsen, S. W. Cambridge MA, MIT Press.

Hadley, R. & Clough, R. (1996) *Care in Chaos: Frustration and Challenge in Community Care*. London, Cassell.

Hamilton, C. (2008) *The Freedom Paradox. Towards a Post-Secular Ethics*. Crows Nest NSW, Allen & Unwin.

Hardina, D. (2004) 'Guidelines for ethical practice in community organization', *Social Work*, 49(4), pp. 595–604.

Healy, K. (2005) *Social Work Theories in Context: Creating Frameworks for Practice*. Basingstoke, Palgrave-Macmillan.

Healy, K. & Meagher, G. (2004) 'The reprofessionalization of social work: collaborative approaches for achieving professional recognition', *British Journal of Social Work*, 34(2), pp. 243–260.

Healy, L. M. (2007) 'Universalism and relativism in social work ethics', *International Social Work*, 50(1), pp. 11–26.

Healy, L. M. (2008) *International Social Work: Professional Action in an Interdependent World*. 2nd Edition. New York, Oxford University Press.

Hikoyeda, N. & Wallace, S. P. (2002) 'Do ethnic-specific long term care facilities improve residents' quality of life? Findings from the Japanese American community', *Journal of Gerontological Social Work*, 36(1–2), pp. 83–106.

Hinman, L. M. (2008) *Ethics: a Pluralistic Approach to Moral Theory*, 4th Edition. Belmont CA, Thomson Higher Education.

Hodge, D. R. & Limb, G. E. (2010) 'Conducting spiritual assessments with Native Americans: enhancing cultural competency in social work practice courses', *Journal of Social Work Education*, 46(2), pp. 265–284.

Hort, S. E. O. (1997) 'Towards a deresidualization of Swedish child welfare policy and practice?', in Gilbert, N. (ed.) *Combating Child Abuse*. New York, Oxford University Press.

Houston, S. (2009) 'Communication, recognition and social work: aligning the ethical theories of Habermas and Honneth', *British Journal of Social Work*, 39(7), pp. 1274–1290.

Howe, D. (2005) *Child Abuse and Neglect: Attachment, Development and Intervention*. Basingstoke, Palgrave-Macmillan.

Howe, D., Brandon, M., Hining, D. & Schofield, G. (1999) *Attachment Theory, Child Maltreatment and Family Support*. Basingstoke, Macmillan.

Hughes, M. & Heycox, K. (2010) *Older People, Ageing and Social Work: Knowledge for Practice*. Crows Nest NSW, Allen & Unwin.

Hugman, R. (1991) *Power in Caring Professions*. London, Macmillan.

Hugman, R. (1998) *Social Welfare and Social Value*. Basingstoke, Macmillan.

Hugman, R. (2005) *New Approaches in Ethics for the Caring Professions*. Basingstoke, Palgrave-Macmillan.

Hugman, R. (2008) 'Ethics in a world of difference', *Ethics & Social Welfare*, 2(2), pp. 118–132.

Hugman, R. (2009) 'But is it social work? Some reflections on mistaken identities', *British Journal of Social Work*, 39(6), pp. 1138–1153.

Hugman, R. (2010) *Understanding International Social Work: a Critical Analysis*. Basingstoke, Palgrave-Macmillan.

Hugman, R. & Smith, D. (1995) 'Ethical issues in social work: an introduction' in Hugman, R. & Smith, D. (eds) *Ethical Issues in Social Work*. London, Routledge.

Hugman, R., Nguyen Thi Thai Lan & Nguyen Thuy Hong (2007) 'Professionalizing social work in Vietnam', *International Social Work*, 50(2), pp. 197–211.

Husband, C. (1995) 'The morally active practitioner and the ethics of anti-racist social work', in Hugman, R. & Smith, D. (eds) *Ethical Issues in Social Work*. London, Routledge.

Ibanez, E. S., Borrego, J., Pemberton, J. R., Terao, S. (2006) 'Cultural factors in decision making about child abuse: indentifying reporter characteristics influencing reporting tendencies', *Child Abuse & Neglect*, 30, pp. 1365–1379.

Ife, J. (2008) *Human Rights and Social Work*. 2nd Edition. Melbourne, Cambridge University Press.

Ife, J. (2009) *Human Rights From Below: Achieving Rights Through Community Development*. Melbourne, Cambridge University Press.

Ife, J. (2010) 'Human rights and social justice', in Gray, M. & Webb, S. A. (eds) *Ethics and Value Perspectives in Social Work*. Basingstoke, Palgrave Macmillan

International Association of Schools of Social Work [IASSW]/International Federation of Social Workers [IFSW] (2004) *Global Standards on Education and Training in Social Work*. Electronic document, downloaded on 11 May 2012 from http://ifsw.org/policies/global-standards.

International Council of Nursing [ICN] (2006) *The ICN Code of Ethics for Nurses*. Geneva, ICN.

International Federation of Social Workers [IFSW] (2011) *IFSW Member Organizations*. Electronic document, downloaded on 1 February 2011 from www.ifsw.org/f38000017.html.

International Federation of Social Workers [IFSW]/International Association of Schools of Social Work [IASSW] (2000/2001) *Definition of Social Work*. Electronic document, downloaded on 1 February 2011 from www.ifsw.org/f38000138.html.

International Federation of Social Workers [IFSW]/International Association of Schools of Social Work [IASSW] (2004) *Ethics in Social Work: Statement of Principles*. Electronic document, downloaded on 1 February 2011 from www.ifsw.org/f38000032.html.

International Union of Psychological Science [IUPS] (2008) *Universal Declaration of Ethical Principles for Psychologists*. Electronic document, downloaded on 23 February 2011 from www.iupsys.net/index.php/ethics/declaration.

Irvine, D. (2001) 'Doctors in the UK: their new professionalism and its regulatory framework', *The Lancet*, 358(9295), pp. 1807–1810.

Jackson, D. (1995) 'Nursing texts and lesbian contexts: lesbian imagery in the nursing literature', *Australian Journal of Advanced Nursing*, 13(1), pp. 25–31.

Jenks, C. (1993) *Culture*. London, Routledge.

Jenks, C. (1996) *Childhood*. London, Routledge.

Johnson, T. J. (1972) *Professions and Power*. London, Macmillan.

Jolley, M. (1989) 'The professionalization of nursing: the uncertain path', in Jolley, M. & Allan, P. (eds) *Current Issues in Nursing*. London, Chapman & Hall.

Jorgensen, A. K. & Rice, J. (2010) 'Urban slum growth and human health: a panel study of infant and child mortality in less-developed countries, 1990–2005', *Journal of Poverty*, 14(4), pp. 382–402.

Joseph, J. & Joseph, H. (2008) 'Ethics for social workers in the era of globalization', *Indian Journal of Social Work*, 69(2), pp. 271–287.

Kant, I. (1964 [1785]) *The Moral Law: Groundwork of the Metaphysics of Morals*. Trans. Paton, H. J. London and New York, Routledge.

Kaseke, E. (2005) 'Social security and older people: an African perspective', *International Social Work*, 48(1), pp. 89–98.

Kekes, J. (1993) *The Morality of Pluralism*. Princeton NJ, Princeton University Press.

Keown, D. (2007) 'Are there "human rights" in Buddhism?', in Bilimoria, P., Prahbu, J. & Sharma, R. (eds) *Indian Ethics: Classical Traditions and Contemporary Challenges, Volume 1*. Aldershot, Ashgate.

Koehn, D. (1994) *The Ground of Professional Ethics*. London, Routledge.

Kolm, R. (1978) 'Ethnicity in social work', *Journal of Religion & Spirituality in Social Work: Social Thought*, 4(1), pp. 3–14.

Koyano, W. (2000) 'Filial piety, co-residence and intergenerational solidarity in Japan', in Liu, W. T. & Kendig, H. (eds) *Who Should Care for the Elderly? East-West Perspectives*. Singapore, Singapore University Press/World Scientific Publishing Co.

Kriz, K. & Skivenes, M. (2010) '"We have very different positions on some issues": how child welfare workers in Norway and England bridge cultural differences when communicating with ethnic minority families', *European Journal of Social Work*, 13(1), pp. 3–18.

Kuper, A. (1999) *Culture: the Anthropologists' Account*. Cambridge MA, Harvard University Press.

Kymlicka, W. (1989) *Liberalism, Community and Culture*. Oxford, The Clarendon Press.

Kymlicka, W. (1995) *Multicultural Citizenship*. Oxford, The Clarendon Press.

Kymlicka, W. (1997) *States, Nations and Cultures*. Assen, van Gorcum.

Lai, K. (2006) *Learning from Chinese Philosophies: Ethics of Interdependent and Contextualized Self*. Aldershot, Ashgate.

Lalor, K. (2004) 'Child sexual abuse in Tanzania and Kenya', *Child Abuse & Neglect*, 28(8), pp. 833–844.

Langan, M. & Day, L. (eds) (1992) *Women, Oppression and Social Work: Issues in Anti-Discriminatory Practice*. London, Routledge.

Lau, A. & Zane, N. (2000) 'Examining the effects of ethnic specific services: an analysis of cost-utilization and treatment outcomes for Asian Americans', *Journal of Community Psychiatry*, 28(1), pp. 63–77.

Leicht, K. T., Walter, T., Sainsaulieu, I. & Davies, C. (2009) 'New public management and new professionalism across nations and contexts', *Current Sociology*, 57(4), pp. 581–605.

Leung, P. P. Y., Chan, C. L. W., Ng, S. M. & Lee, M. Y. (2009) 'Towards mind-body-spirit integration: East meets West in clinical social work practice', *Smith College Studies in Social Work*, 80(2–3), pp. 215–227.

Leung, T. T. F. (2010) 'Social work professionalism in self-help organizations', *International Social Work*, 53(4), pp. 474–488.

Liberman, A. (2010) *Women in Social Work Who Have Changed the World*. Chicago, Lyceum Books.

Liljegren, A., Delgran, P. & Höjer, S. (2008) 'The heroine and the capitalist: the profession's debate about privatization of Swedish social work', *European Journal of Social Work*, 11(3), pp. 195–208.

Lin, W.-I. & Wang, K. Y.-T. (2010) 'What does professionalization mean? Tracing the trajectory of social work education in Taiwan', *Social Work Education*, 29(8), pp. 869–881.

Lloyd, L. (2010) 'The individual in social care: the ethics of care and the "personalization agenda" of services for older people in England', *Ethics & Social Welfare*, 4(2), pp. 188–200.

Lombard, A. & Kruger, E. (2009) 'Older persons: the case of South Africa', *Ageing International*, 34, pp. 119–135.

Lonne, B., Mcdonald, C. & Fox, T. (2004) 'Ethical practice in the contemporary human services', *Journal of Social Work*, 4(3), pp. 345–367.

Lum, T. Y. (2005) 'Understanding the racial and ethnic differences in caregiving arrangements', *Journal of Gerontological Social Work*, 45(4), pp. 3–21.

Lundy, C. (2004) *Social Work and Social Justice*. Calgary, Broadview Press.

Lundy, C. (2006) 'Social work's commitment to social and economic justice: a challenge to the profession', in Hall, N. (ed.) *Social Work: Making a Difference. Social Work Around the World IV*. Berne/Oslo, IFSW/FAFO.

Lymbery, M. (2007) 'Social work in its organizational context', in Lymbery, M. & Postle, K. (eds) *Social Work: a Companion to Learning*. London, Sage.

Lyons, K., Manion, K. & Carlsen, M. (2006) *International Perspectives in Social Work: Global Conditions and Local Practices*. Basingstoke, Palgrave-Macmillan.

Macdonald, G. & Macdonald, K. (1995) 'Ethical issues in social work research', in Hugman, R. & Smith, D. (eds) *Ethical Issues in Social Work*. London, Routledge.

MacIntyre, A. (1983) *After Virtue: a Study in Moral Theory*. London, Duckworth.

MacIntyre, A. (1998) *A Short History of Ethics*. 2nd Edition. London, Routledge.

MacLeod, M. (1999) 'The abuse of children in institutional settings: children's perspectives', in Stanely, N., Manthorpe, J. & Penhale, B. (eds) *Institutional Abuse: Perspectives Across the Life Course*. London, Routledge.

Mafile'o, T. (2004) 'Exploring Tongan social work: *fakafekau'aki* (connecting) and *fakatokilalo* (humility)', *Qualitative Social Work*, 3(3), pp. 239–257.

Mafile'o, T. (2006) '*Matakainga* (behaving like family): the social worker-client relationship in Pasifika social work', *Social Work Review/Tu Mau*, 18(1), pp. 31–36.

Maglajlic, R. A. (2011) 'International organizations, social work and war: a "frog's perspective" on the bird's eye view', in Lavalette, M. & Ioakimidis, V. (eds) *Social Work in Extremis*. Bristol, The Policy Press.

Maidment, J. (2006) 'The quiet remedy: a dialogue on reshaping professional relationships', *Families in Society: the Journal of Contemporary Human Services*, 87(1), pp. 115–121.

Maslow, A. (1970) *Motivation and Personality*. 2nd Edition. New York, Harper & Row.

McAuliffe, D. & Chenoweth, L. (2008) 'Leave no stone unturned: the inclusive model of ethical decision making', *Ethics & Social Welfare*, 2(1), pp. 38–49.

McBeath, G. & Webb, S. A. (2002) 'Virtue ethics and social work: being lucky, realistic and not doing one's duty', *British Journal of Social Work*, 32(8), pp.1015–1036.

McFayden, A. (2002) 'Secular public theology', *Crucible: The Journal of the Church of England Board of Social Responsibility*, July–September, pp. 131–138.

McLeod, M. (1999) 'The abuse of children in institutional settings: children's perspectives', in Stanely, N., Manthorpe, J. & Penhale, B. (eds) *Institutional Abuse: Perspectives Across the Life-Course*. London, Routledge.

McMahon, A. (2005) 'Social work practice in an ethnically and culturally diverse Australia', in Alston, M. & McKinnon, J. (eds) *Social Work: Fields of Practice*. South Melbourne, Oxford University Press.

Mehta, K. (2006) 'A critical review of Singapore's policies aimed at supporting families caring for older members', *Aging & Social Policy*, 18(3), pp. 43–57.

Mendes, P. (2002) 'Social workers and the ethical dilemmas of community action campaigns: lessons from the Australian state of Victoria', *Community Development Journal*, 37(2), pp. 157–166.

Midgley, J. (1981) *Professional Imperialism*. London, Heinemann.

Midgley, J. & Sanzenbach, P. (1989) 'Social work, religion and the global challenge of fundamentalism', *International Social Work*, 32(4), pp. 273–287.

Mill, J. S. (1910 [1861]) *Utilitarianism, Liberty & Representative Government*. London/ New York, J. M. Dent & Sons/E. P. Dutton.

Mjelde-Mossey, L. A., Chi, I. & Lou, V. W. Q. (2005) 'Assessing tradition in Chinese elders living in a socially changing environment', *Journal of Human Behavior in the Social Environment*, 11(3), pp. 41–47.

Modood, T. (2007) *Multiculturalism*. Cambridge, Polity Press.

Mohanty, J. N. (2007) 'Dharma, imperatives and tradition: towards an Indian theory of moral action', in Bilimoria, P., Prabhu, J. & Sharma, R. (eds) *Indian Ethics: Classical Traditions and Contemporary Challenges*. Aldershot, Ashgate.

Moonie, N., Bates A. & Spencer-Perkins, D. (2004) *Diversity and Rights in Care*. London, Heinemann.

Morris, P. M. (2002) 'The capabilities perspective: a framework for social justice', *Families in Society: the Journal of Contemporary Human Services*, 83(4), pp. 365–373.

Morrison, E. E. (ed.) (2009) *Health Care Ethics: Critical Issues for the 21st Century*. 2nd Edition. Sudbury MA, Jones and Bartlett Publishers.

Morse, C. A. & Messimeri-Kianidis, V. (2002) 'Keeping it in the family', *Social Work in Health Care*, 34(3–4), pp. 299–314.

Munford, R. & Walsh-Tapiata, W. (2006) 'Community development: working in the bicultural context of Aotearoa New Zealand', *Community Development Journal*, 41(4), pp. 426–442.

Murphy, T. (2011) 'Social work and social development in Central Asia', in Lavalette, M. & Ioakimidis, V. (eds) *Social Work in Extremis*. Bristol, The Policy Press.

Nagel, A. K. (2006) 'Charitable Choice: the religious dimension of the US welfare-reform – theoretical and methodological reflections on "faith-based organizations" as social service agencies', *Numen*, 53(1), pp. 78–111.

Nagel, T. (1979) *Mortal Questions*. Cambridge, Cambridge University Press.

National Association of Social Workers [NASW] (2008) *Code of Ethics*. Washington DC, NASW.

Neocleous, G. (2011) 'Social welfare to protect elderly victims of war in Cyprus', in Lavalette, M. & Ioakimidis, V. (eds) *Social Work in Extremis*. Bristol, The Policy Press.

Nguyen Thi Thai Lan (2011) 'Vietnam: commentary', in Banks, S. & Nøhr, K. (eds) *Practising Social Work Ethics Around the World: Cases and Commentaries*. London, Taylor & Francis.

Nimmagadda, J. & Cowger, C. D. (1999) 'Cross-cultural practice: social worker ingenuity in the indigenization of practice knowledge', *International Social Work*, 42(3), pp. 261–276.

Noble, C. (2004) 'Social work education, training and standards in the Asia-Pacific region', *Social Work Education*, 23(5), pp. 527–536.

Nussbaum, M. (1998) 'Public philosophy and international feminism', *Ethics*, 108(4), pp. 762–796.

Nussbaum, M. (2000) *Women and Human Development*. Cambridge, Cambridge University Press.

Nussbaum, M. (2001) *Upheavals of Thought*. Cambridge, Cambridge University Press.

Nussbaum, M. (2002) 'Capabilities and social justice', *International Studies Review*, 4(2), pp. 123–135.

Nussbaum, M. (2006) *Frontiers of Justice: Disability, Nationality, Species Membership*. Cambridge MA, Belknap/Harvard University Press.

O'Connor, I., Hughes, M., Turney, D., Wilson, J. & Setterlund, D. (2006) *Social Work and Social Care Practice*. London, Sage.

O'Hagan, K. (2001) *Cultural Competence in the Caring Professions*. London, Jessica Kingsley.

O'Neill, O. (2005) 'The dark side of human rights', *International Affairs*, 81(2), pp. 427–439.

Oliver, M. (1990) *The Politics of Disablement*. London, Macmillan.

Olson, J. (2007) 'Social work's professional and social justice projects: conflicts in discourse', *Journal of Progressive Human Services*, 18(1), pp. 45–69.

Osei-Hwedie, K. (1993) 'The challenge of social work in Africa: starting the indigenization process', *Journal of Social Development in Africa*, 8(1), pp. 19–30.

Osei-Hwedie, K., Ntseane, D. & Jacques, G. (2006) 'Searching for appropriateness in social work education in Botswana', *Social Work Education*, 25(6), pp. 569–590.

Øvretveit, J., Mathias, P. & Thompson, T. (1997) *Interprofessional Working for Health and Social Care*. Basingstoke, Palgrave Macmillan.

Ozmete, E. (2009) 'The core life values as viewed by Turkish women', *Indian Journal of Social Work*, 70(1), pp. 85–102.

Parekh, B. (2010) *Gandhi: a Brief Insight*. New York, Sterling Publishing Co.

Parrott, L. (2010) *Values and Ethics in Social Work Practice*. 2nd Edition. London, Learning Matters.

Parton, N. (2003) 'Rethinking *professional* practice: the contributions of social constructionism and the feminist "ethics of care"', *British Journal of Social Work*, 33(1), pp. 1–16.

Parton, N. (2009) 'Challenges to practice and knowledge in child welfare social work: from the "social" to the "informational"?', *Children and Youth Services Review*, 31, pp. 715–721.

Patel, L. (2005) *Social Welfare and Social Development in South Africa*. Cape Town, Oxford University Press.

Payne, M. (2005) *The Origins of Social Work*. Basingstoke, Palgrave-Macmillan.

Payne, M. & Askeland, G. A. (2008) *Globalization and International Social Work: Postmodern Change and Challenge*. Aldershot, Ashgate.

Peter, T. (2009) 'Exploring taboos: comparing male- and female-perpetrated child sexual abuse', *Journal of Interpersonal Violence*, 24(7), pp. 1111–1128.

Pierce, L. H. & Bozalek, V. (2004) 'Child abuse in South Africa: an examination of how child abuse and neglect are defined', *Child Abuse & Neglect*, 27, pp. 817–832.

Pierce, L. H. & Bozalek, V. (2009) 'Collaboration for the promotion of community of community and individual health', *Social Work in Public Health*, 24(1–2), pp. 117–123.

Pittaway, E., Bartolomei, L. & Rees, S. (2007) 'Gendered dimensions of the 2004 tsunami and a potential social work response in post-disaster situations', *International Social Work*, 50(3) pp. 307–319.

Pizzey, E. (1974) *Scream Quietly or the Neighbours Will Hear*. Harmondsworth, Penguin.

Postle, K. & Beresford, P. (2007) 'Capacity building and the reconception of political participation: a role for social care workers?', *British Journal of Social Work*, 37(1), pp. 143–158.

Rachels, J. (1998) *Ethical Theory*. New York, Oxford University Press.

Rachels, J. (2003) *The Elements of Moral Philosophy*, 4th Edition. New York, McGraw-Hill.

Radermacher, H., Feldman, S. & Browning, C. (2009) 'Mainstream versus ethno-specific community aged care services: it's not an "either or"', *Australasian Journal on Ageing*, 28(2), pp. 58–63.

Rainbow Spirit Elders (2007) *Rainbow Spirit Theology: Towards an Australian Aboriginal Theology*. Hindmarsh, ATF Press.

Rawls, J. (1972) *A Theory of Justice*. Oxford, The Clarendon Press.

Razack, N. (2000) 'North/South collaborations', *Journal of Progressive Human Services*, 11(1), pp. 71–91.

Reamer, F. G. (1999) *Social Work Values and Ethics*. 2nd Edition. New York, Columbia University Press.

Reingold, D. A., Pirog, M. & Brady, D. (2007) 'Empirical evidence on faith-based organizations in an era of welfare reform', *Social Services Review*, 81(2), pp. 245–283.

Reisch, M. (2002) 'Defining social justice in a socially unjust world', *Families in Society: the Journal of Contemporary Human Services*, 83(4), pp. 343–354.

Reisch, M. (2008) 'From melting pot to multiculturalism: the impact of racial and ethnic diversity on social work and social justice in the USA', *British Journal of Social Work*, 38(4), pp. 788–804.

Reisch, M. & Andrews, J. (2002) *The Road Not Taken: a History of Radical Social Work in the United States*. New York, Brunner-Routledge.

Reisch, M. & Lowe, J. I. (2000) '"Of means and ends" revisited: teaching ethical community organizing in an unethical society', *Journal of Community Practice*, 7(1), pp. 19–38.

Rhee, S., Chang, J. & Youn, S. (2003) 'Korean American pastors' perceptions and attitudes towards child abuse', *Journal of Ethnic and Cultural Diversity in Social Work*, 12(1), pp. 27–46.

Ritzer, G. (2000) *The McDonaldization of Society*, 3rd Edition. Thousand Oaks CA, Pine Forge.

Roberts, J. V. (2000) 'Changing public attitudes towards corporal punishment: the effects of statutory reform in Sweden', *Child Abuse & Neglect*, 24(8), pp. 1027–1035.

Robinson, L. (1995) *Psychology for Social Workers: Black Perspectives*. London, Routledge.

Robinson, L. (2007) *Cross-cultural Child Development for Social Workers: an Introduction*. Basingstoke, Palgrave Macmillan.

Rorty, R. (1999) *Philosophy and Social Hope*. London, Penguin Books.

Ross, E. (2008) 'The intersection of cultural practices and ethics in a rights-based society: implications for South African social workers', *International Social Work*, 51(3), pp. 384–395.

Sakamoto, I. & Pitner, R. O. (2005) 'Use of critical consciousness in anti-oppressive social work practice: disentangling power dynamics at personal and structural levels', *British Journal of Social Work*, 35(4), pp. 435–452.

Saldov, M. & Kakai, H. (2004) 'The ethics of medical decision-making with Japanese-American elders in Hawai'i', *Journal of Human Behavior in the Social Environment*, 10(1), pp. 113–130.

Sanyal, I. (2010) 'Varña and Jāti', in Sanyal, I. & Sashinungla (eds) *Ethics and Culture: Some Indian Reflections*. New Delhi, Decent Books.

Scourfield, P. (2007) 'Social care and the modern citizen: client, consumer, service user, manager and entrepreneur', *British Journal of Social Work*, 37, pp. 107–122.

Sen, A. (1985) *Commodities and Capabilities*. Amsterdam/New York, Elsevier Science Publishing Company.

Sen, A. (1999) *Development as Freedom*. Oxford, Oxford University Press.

Sen, A. (2004) *Rationality and Freedom*. Cambridge MA, Harvard University Press.

Sercombe, H. (2010) *Youth Work Ethics*. London, Sage.

Sewpaul, V. (2007) 'Challenging East-West value dichotomies and essentialising discourse on culture and social work', *International Journal of Social Welfare*, 16(4), pp. 398–407.

Shardlow, S. (ed.) (1989) *The Values of Change in Social Work*. London, Routledge.

Siderits, M. (2007) 'Buddhist Reductionism and the structure of Buddhist ethics', in Bilimoria, P., Prabhu, J. & Sharma, R. (eds) *Indian Ethics: Classical Traditions and Contemporary Challenges*. Aldershot, Ashgate.

Silavwe, G. (1995) 'The need for a new social work perspective in an African setting: the case of social casework in Zambia', *British Journal of Social Work*, 25(1), pp. 71–84.

Singer, P. (2002) *One World: the Ethics of Globalization*. Melbourne, Text Publishing.

Smith, D. (ed.) (2004) *Social Work and Evidence-Based Practice*. London, Jessica Kingsley.

Solas, J. (2008) 'Social work and social justice: what are we fighting for?', *Australian Social Work*, 61(2), pp. 124–136.

Solomon, B. B. (1976) *Black Empowerment: Social Work With Oppressed Communities*. New York, Columbia University Press.

Soydan, H. (2010) 'Anti-racist ethics', in Gray, M. & Webb, S. A. (eds) *Ethics and Value Perspectives in Social Work*. Basingstoke, Palgrave-Macmillan.

Spira, M. & Wall, J. (2009) 'Cultural and intergenerational narratives: understanding responses to elderly family members in declining health', *Journal of Gerontological Social Work*, 52(2), pp. 105–123.

Stark, C. (2010) 'The neoliberal ideology and the challenges for social work ethics and practice', *Revista de Asistenta Sociala*, 1, pp. 9–19.

Stubbs, P. (1985) 'The employment of Black social workers: from "ethnic sensitivity" to anti-racism', *Critical Social Policy*, 4(3), pp. 6–27.

Svensson, L. G (2006) 'New professionalism, trust and competence', *Current Sociology*, 54(4), 579–593.

Taylor, C. (1994) 'The politics of recognition', in Gutmann, A. (ed.) *Multiculturalism: Examining the Politics of Recognition*. Princeton NJ, The Princeton University Press.

Taylor, C. and White, S. (2001) 'Knowledge, truth and reflexivity: the problem of judgement', *Journal of Social Work*, 1(1), pp. 37–59.

Taylor, C. and White, S. (2006) 'Knowledge and reasoning in social work: educating for humane judgement', *British Journal of Social Work*, 36(6), pp. 937–954.

Templeman, S. B. (2004) 'Social work in the new Russia at the start of the millennium', *International Social Work*, 47(1), pp. 95–107.

Thompson, N. (1993) *Anti-Discriminatory Practice*. Basingstoke, Macmillan.

Thyer, B. A. (2007) 'Social work education and clinical learning: towards evidence-based practice?', *Clinical Social Work Journal*, 35, pp. 25–32.

Tien, W. Y. M., David, M. K. & Alagappar, P. (2009) 'Filial responsibility among Malaysian youth towards elderly parents', *Indian Journal of Social Work*, 70(4), pp. 647–663.

Timms, N. (1983) *Social Work Values: an Inquiry*. London, Routledge & Kegan Paul.

Tiwari, A. (2007) 'Human rights violations against Dalits: a case of failed state?', *Indian Journal of Social Work*, 68(1), pp. 73–87.

Toren, N. (1972) *Social Work: the Case of a Semi-Profession*. London, Sage.

Tronto, J. (1993) *Moral Boundaries: a Political Argument for an Ethic of Care*. New York, Routledge.

Tsang, A. K. T., Sin, R., Jia, C. & Yan, M. C. (2008) 'Another snapshot of social work in China: capturing multiple positioning and interesting discourses in rapid movement', *Australian Social Work*, 61(1), pp. 72–87.

Tsui, M. S. & Chan, K. H. R. (1995) 'Divergence and convergence: in search of a common base of the notion of the welfare state in China and in the West', *Journal of Comparative Social Welfare*, 11(1), pp. 42–55.

United Nations [UN] (1948) *Universal Declaration of Human Rights*. New York, United Nations.

United Nations Development Program [UNDP] (2004) *Human Development Report 2004: Cultural Liberty in Today's Diverse World*. New York, UNDP.

Versfeld, M. (2005) *The Philosopher's Cookbook*. Sydney, Figment Publishing.

Walton, R. & El Nasr, M. M. A. (1988) 'The indigenization and authentization of social work in Egypt', *The Community Development Journal*, 2393), pp. 148–155.

Walzer, M. (1994) *Thick and Thin: Morality at Home and Abroad*. Notre Dame IN, University of Notre Dame Press.

Warburton, J., Bartlett, H. & Rao, V. (2009) 'Ageing and cultural diversity: policy and practice issues', *Australian Social Work*, 62(2), pp. 168–185.

Weaver, H. N. (2004) 'The elements of cultural competence', *Journal of Ethnic and Cultural Diversity in Social Work*, 13(1), pp. 19–35.

Webb, S. A. (2009) 'Against difference and diversity in social work: the case of human rights', *International Journal of Social Welfare*, 18(3), pp. 307–316.

Webb, S. A. (2010) 'Virtue ethics', in Gray, M. & Webb, S. A. (eds) *Ethics and Value Perspectives in Social Work*. Basingstoke, Palgrave-Macmillan.

Webb, S. A. & McBeath, G. (1989) 'A political critique of Kantian ethics in social work', *British Journal of Social Work*, 19(6), pp. 491–506.

Webster, P. (2010) 'Codes of conduct', in Gray, M. & Webb, S. A. (eds) *Ethics and Value Perspectives in Social Work*. Basingstoke, Palgrave-Macmillan.

Webster, Y. O. (2002) 'A human-centric alternative to diversity and multicultural education', *Journal of Social Work Education*, 38(1), pp. 17–36.

Weeks, W. (1995) 'Women's work, the gendered division of labour and community services', in Weeks, W. & Wilson, J. (eds) *Issues Facing Australian Families: Human Services Respond*. Melbourne, Longman.

Weiss, I. (2005) 'Is there a global common core to social work? A cross-national comparative study of BSW graduates', *Social Work*, 50(2), pp. 101–110.

Weiss-Gal, I. & Welbourne, P. (2008) 'The professionalization of social work: a cross-national exploration', *International Journal of Social Welfare*, 17(4), pp. 281–290.

Westermark, E. (1932) *Ethical Relativity*. London, Kegan Paul, Trench, Trubner & Co.

Whiting, R. (2008) '"No room for religion or spirituality or cooking tips": exploring practical atheism as an unspoken consensus in the development of social work values in England', *Ethics & Social Welfare*, 2(1), pp. 67–83.

Whitney, S. D., Tajima, E. J., Herrenkohl, T. I. & Huang, B. (2006) 'Defining child abuse: exploring difference in ratings of discipline severity among child welfare practitioners', *Child and Adolescent Social Work Journal*, 23(3), pp. 316–342.

Wilding, P. (1982) *Social Welfare and Professional Power*. London, Routledge.

Williams, B. (1972) *Morality: an Introduction to Ethics*. Cambridge, Cambridge University Press.

Williams, B. (1981) *Moral Luck. Philosophical Papers 1973–1980*. Cambridge, Cambridge University Press.

Williams, B. (1985) *Ethics and the Limits of Philosophy*. London, Fontana/Collins.

Williams, C. & Soydan, H. (2005) 'When and how does ethnicity matter? A cross-national study of social work responses to ethnicity in child protection cases', *British Journal of Social Work*, 35(6), pp. 901–920.

Willumsen, E. & Skivenes, M. (2005) 'Collaboration between service users and professionals: legitimate decisions in child protection – a Norwegian model', *Child & Family Social Work*, 10, pp. 197–206.

Winter, B., Thompson, D. & Jeffreys, S. (2002) 'The UN approach to harmful traditional practices', *International Feminist Journal of Politics*, 4(1), pp. 72–94.

Witz, A. (1992) *Patriarchy and the Professions*. London, Routledge.

World Medical Association [WMA] (2005) *Medical Ethics Manual*. Ferney-Voltaire, WMA.

Yan, M. C. (2008) 'Exploring cultural tensions in cross-cultural social work practice', *Social Work*, 53(4), pp. 317–328.

Yan, M. C. & Cheung, K. W. (2006) 'The politics of indigenization: a case study of development of social work in China', *Journal of Sociology and Social Welfare*, 33(2), pp. 63–84.

Yellow Bird, M. J. (1999) 'Indian, American Indian and Native American: counterfeit identities', *Winds of Change: a Magazine for American Indian Education and Opportunity*, 14(1). Electronic document downloaded on 8 June 2011 from www.aistm.org/yellowbirdessay.htm.

Yellow Bird, M. & Gray, M. (2008) 'Indigenous people and the language of social work', in Gray, M., Coates, J. & Yellow Bird, M. (eds) *Indigenous Social Work Around the World: Towards Culturally Relevant Education and Practice*. Aldershot, Ashgate.

Yip, K. S. (2004) 'A Chinese cultural critique of the global qualifying standards for social work education', *Social Work Education*, 23(5), pp. 597–612.

Youth Affairs Council of Western Australia [YACWA] (2003) *Code of Ethics*. West Leederville, YACWA.

Yuen-Tsang, A. W. K. & Sung, P. P. L. (2002) 'Capacity building through networking: integrating professional knowledge with indigenous practice', in Tan, N. T. & Dodds, I. (eds) *Social Work Around the World II*. Berne, IFSW Press.

Zawati, H. M. (2007) 'Impunity or immunity: wartime male rape and sexual torture as a crime against humanity', *Torture*, 17(1), pp. 27–47.

Index

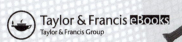